Everything

You Need

To Know

Forensic Nurse

ALEXANDRE CAREWELL

2

Table of contents

« In the interwoven webs of forensic medicine, each clue is a whisper of truth, giving a voice to those who can no longer speak, and illuminating justice in the darkness of doubt. »

INTRODUCTION

Introduction to forensic medicine

At the crossroads of medical science and law, forensic medicine is emerging as a fascinating discipline which, over the centuries, has continually evolved to meet the demands of a justice system in constant search of the truth. Not only is forensic medicine the science of determining the cause of death, it also plays a crucial role in identifying victims, detecting crimes and providing evidence in legal proceedings.

Forensic medicine is not confined to the cold confines of a morgue; it is deployed throughout the fabric of society, dealing with situations as varied as road accidents, unexplained deaths in the home and crime. The unique feature of this discipline is that it combines scientific rigour with profound humanity. Indeed, each case studied takes on a singular importance, constantly reminding professionals in the field that behind each sample, each swab, lies a story, a life.

The essence of forensic medicine goes far beyond the simple autopsy. It encompasses a multitude of specialities ranging from toxicology to forensic anthropology, from ballistics to genetics. Each branch offers a different perspective, but all converge towards the same goal: to understand, explain and provide answers.

These answers are often eagerly awaited, both by bereaved families and by the judicial authorities. They can shed light on, and even resolve, complex criminal cases. The role of forensic medicine does not stop at establishing evidence or finding the truth. It also plays a preventive role, identifying patterns or trends that could, over time, help reduce certain types of death or trauma.

It is therefore essential to recognise that forensic medicine, although often perceived as a gloomy discipline, is a fundamental pillar of our judicial and social system. It is the silent guardian of the stories that the disappeared can no longer tell, and through its prism, justice can be dispensed with clarity, precision and humanity.

The role of the nurse
in forensic medicine

Although forensic medicine is immediately associated with emblematic figures such as the forensic pathologist or the investigator, there are some lesser-known but equally essential players among its ranks: the nurses. Nurses are health professionals with solid medical training, the ability to adapt and a keen sense of observation, and they play a pivotal role in forensic teams.

At first glance, one might wonder about the exact role of a nurse in a field where autopsies and post-mortem analyses predominate. However, it is important to understand that forensic medicine is not just about studying the deceased. It also takes an interest, and sometimes a very strong one, in the living: victims of assault or abuse, or witnesses requiring specific care and forensic sampling. In this context, nurses often become the first point of contact, providing clinical expertise and invaluable human support.

Post-mortem nurses work closely with the forensic pathologist, particularly during autopsies. They prepare the body, assist with the examination, manage the samples and ensure that they are traceable. This inter-professional collaboration ensures that procedures are carried out with the utmost scientific rigour, while respecting the dignity of the deceased.

In addition, forensic nurses often receive in-depth training to meet specific needs. This may include caring for victims of sexual violence, taking specific forensic samples or accompanying people in a state of shock or distress.

Beyond these technical skills, the forensic nurse is often a pillar of emotional support. Whether for a bereaved family, a traumatised victim or even other members of the forensic team, their ability to listen, reassure and guide is crucial. He embodies that touch of humanity at the heart of a world where science and justice predominate.

Finally, the constant evolution of forensic medicine, with the emergence of new techniques and technologies, offers nurses opportunities for specialisation and professional development. Whether they are on the front line at crime scenes, in analysis laboratories or at the bedside of victims, their role is central, making them key players in the quest for truth and justice that forensic medicine embodies.

Chapter 1:
HISTORY AND FOUNDATIONS
FORENSIC MEDICINE

Origins and historical development forensic medicine

The marriage between medicine and the law is nothing new. Indeed, the interaction between these two worlds goes back to ancient times, long before forensic medicine was given a name and formal recognition.

The earliest traces of forensic medicine can be found in ancient civilisations such as Egypt, Greece and China. Egyptian papyri dating back several millennia before our era already describe post-mortem examinations carried out to understand the cause of death. In China, during the Song dynasty, a treatise called "Washing Away of Wrongs" was written, setting out methods for determining the cause of death, echoing our modern autopsies.

The Greco-Roman world, for its part, was distinguished by its rational approach to medicine and the importance attached to medical evidence in court cases. Hippocrates, the father of modern medicine, himself spoke of the importance of the doctor's role in providing legal evidence.

However, the real development of forensic medicine as a structured discipline coincided with the evolution of scientific thought during the Renaissance. Advances in anatomy, thanks to figures such as Vesalius and da Vinci, paved the way for a more detailed understanding of the human body. At the same time, the rise of modern judicial systems required greater medical expertise to inform the courts.

The 19th century was a pivotal period. With urbanisation and rapid social change, the need to identify the causes of death, whether natural, accidental or criminal, became crucial. The first chairs of forensic medicine were established in European universities, and toxicology emerged as a major sub-discipline, with scientists such as Mathieu Orfila in France pioneering the detection of poisons.

The 20th century saw forensic medicine grow and diversify. Advances in genetics gave rise to genomic forensics, enabling precise identifications to be made using DNA. Technological advances also brought more sophisticated imaging tools, dating techniques and increasingly advanced laboratory analysis methods.

Today, forensic medicine is a multidisciplinary discipline that continues to evolve. It embraces advances in biotechnology, bioinformatics and artificial intelligence to adapt to the changing needs of society. It is both a witness to the shadows of humanity and a guarantor of justice, a delicate balance inherited from its deep roots and rich, fascinating history.

The importance of forensic medicine in the judicial system

Forensic medicine, with its many facets, is an essential pillar of the modern legal system. It represents the meeting point between medical science and the search for legal truth, providing a bridge between the biological complexity of the human being and society's need for justice.

- **Establishing incontrovertible proof**: At the heart of the legal process, proof is king. And what could be more convincing than tangible evidence rooted in biology or chemistry? Whether through toxicological analyses revealing the presence of illegal substances, post-mortem examinations determining the cause of death or genetic analyses identifying a suspect, forensic medicine provides first-rate evidence.

- **Protecting the innocent**: Paradoxically, the same discipline that can incriminate is also the one that protects. How many innocent people have been exonerated thanks to DNA analysis? Forensic medicine ensures that justice is not only swift, but above all accurate and fair.
- **Caring for victims**: As well as its role in solving crimes, forensic science also has a crucial role to play in caring for living victims, whether they are victims of violence, assault or neglect. Gathering medical evidence, carrying out examinations and taking samples with compassion and professionalism can not only help in the prosecution of criminals, but also offer vital support to victims.
- **Prevention and education**: By studying recurring patterns, whether in deaths linked to overdoses, road accidents or domestic violence, forensic medicine helps to identify trends and inform public policy. It plays a preventive role, providing data that can lead to awareness campaigns, legislative changes or community initiatives.
- **Constantly evolving law**: As science advances, the law must evolve in parallel. The ethical and legal issues raised by advances such as genomics and bioinformatics require an in-depth understanding of the medical implications. Forensic medicine, at the frontier of these advances, guides and informs legislative decisions.

Forensic medicine is much more than just a tool of the justice system: it is one of its cornerstones. By balancing scientific rigour with the imperatives of justice, it ensures

16

that the search for the truth is both precise and humane. Without it, our judicial system would be deprived of one of its most precious resources, losing efficiency, fairness and justice.

The changing role of the nurse in this area

The nurse, often seen as the doctor's faithful shadow, has seen his or her role change dramatically in forensic medicine, as in other medical specialities. This journey through time reveals not only changes in the nursing profession, but also a revolution in the way society perceives and values this crucial health player.

- **From the origins to the modern era**: Historically, the forensic nurse was mainly a technical assistant, helping the medical examiner with his or her tasks, preparing bodies for autopsy or helping with sample management. Although these roles remain fundamental, the profession has undergone a major evolution towards greater autonomy and specialisation.
- **Recognition and specialisation**: Over time, the role of the forensic nurse has expanded. Today, there are specialised training courses offering specific skills in taking forensic samples, treating victims of violence, and providing expertise in fields such as toxicology and genetics. This specialisation has also opened the door to recognition of nurses as experts in their own right, capable of giving evidence in court or conducting research.
- **Beyond technical skills**: The evolution of the nurse's role has not been limited to the acquisition of technical skills. The human aspect of the profession

has become increasingly important. In the delicate context of forensic medicine, where trauma is often omnipresent, the nurse's ability to offer psychological and emotional support has become essential. Nurses are often the first line of contact for victims and their families, playing a crucial role in providing guidance and support.

- **Influencing policies and protocols**: As the profession gained recognition and expertise, forensic nurses also began to influence protocols, standards and guidelines. Their practical, first-hand knowledge of the realities on the ground has positioned them as key players in the development of best practice and recommendations.
- **Leadership and research**: Last but not least, modernity has seen the emergence of forensic nurse researchers and leaders, involved in advanced studies, contributing to the advancement of knowledge in the field and defending the interests of the profession at institutional and legislative levels.

The changing role of the forensic nurse reflects a wider societal shift, recognising the value and expertise of these health professionals. Far from being merely performers, they are now partners, leaders and experts, making an invaluable contribution to the quest for truth and justice inherent in forensic medicine.

Chapter 2:
THE WORKING ENVIRONMENT

The mortuary and autopsy rooms

The mortuary and autopsy room are emblematic elements of forensic medicine. These spaces are charged with emotion, discovery and meticulous scientific research. They represent the frontier where life meets death and where science strives to reveal the mysteries associated with it.

The morgue: Originally, the word "morgue" referred to a room where prisoners were exposed to the public. Today, it refers to the place where the bodies of the deceased are kept before burial or cremation.
* **Main function**: The morgue is mainly used to store bodies in a preserved state, pending identification by the families or autopsy.
* **Preservation technologies**: Over time, preservation methods have evolved. Refrigeration has become the norm, replacing older methods that used ice or chemical substances.

The autopsy room: This is where the body is examined in detail to determine the cause of death.
* **Organisation and equipment**: Designed to facilitate rigorous investigation, it is equipped with stainless steel tables, powerful lighting and a range of specialist surgical instruments. Extraction equipment is also present to remove fumes and odours, ensuring a healthy environment for staff.
* **The autopsy process**: It begins with an external assessment of the body, followed by the opening of the body to examine the internal organs. Each organ is carefully examined, weighed and, if necessary,

samples are taken for further analysis, such as toxicology.

- **Multidisciplinarity**: Although often associated with forensic pathologists, the autopsy room sees the joint work of many professionals: forensic nurses, laboratory technicians, pathologists and sometimes even experts in entomology or anthropology, depending on the nature of the case.
- **Safety and hygiene**: Autopsy rooms must meet strict health and safety standards to protect staff from biological hazards. Personal protective equipment such as gowns, gloves and masks are essential.

The morgue and the autopsy room are not just cold, sterile rooms; they are the theatres of human stories, where each body tells a unique story. Every scar, every wound, every anomaly has a meaning. And it is in these spaces that forensic medicine, with all its know-how and technology, strives to decipher these stories, providing answers for the living and justice for the dead.

Specific equipment forensic medicine

Forensic medicine, as the crossroads between medicine and justice, requires a particularly specialised set of tools and equipment to ensure accurate and reliable analyses. These instruments are essential not only for determining the cause of death, but also for providing evidence in various judicial contexts.

- **Autopsy tables**: Generally made of stainless steel for easy cleaning and disinfection, they are designed with channels to drain fluids and can also be fitted with integrated X-rays.

- **Scalpels and surgical instruments**: Used to open the body and examine internal organs. Some are specifically designed for forensic medicine, such as the autopsy knife or the bone saw.
- **X-ray equipment**: Before opening the body, an X-ray may be taken to detect any foreign objects, fractures or anomalies.
- **Microscopy equipment**: Used to examine samples of tissue or other substances at a microscopic level.
- **Forensic sampling kits**: These kits, often used in cases of sexual assault, contain everything needed to take samples of tissue, fluids and other evidence in a sterile manner.
- **Toxicology equipment**: Used to detect and quantify the presence of medicines, drugs or toxins in body fluids.
- **Photography systems**: High-quality cameras are used to document lesions, tattoos, scars and other relevant body features.
- **Cold rooms**: Located in the mortuary, these are used to store bodies in a preserved state until the autopsy or release of the body.
- **Fingerprint identification systems**: compare the fingerprints of the deceased with databases to facilitate identification.
- **Personal protective equipment (PPE)**: Including gowns, gloves, masks and goggles to ensure the safety of personnel during autopsies and sample handling.
- **DNA analysis kits**: To extract, amplify and analyse DNA for identification purposes or to match it with suspects.
- **Entomological instruments**: In some cases, studying the insects present on a body can provide valuable information about the time and circumstances of death.

All this equipment, combining cutting-edge technology and precision, is crucial to forensic medicine. Each instrument plays a specific role in the search for the truth, helping experts to unravel the mysteries surrounding death, trauma or crime, and ensuring that justice can be done with the greatest possible accuracy.

Precautions
health and safety

When we think of forensic medicine, we often think of the legal or scientific aspects, but an equally crucial aspect is that of safety and hygiene. The delicate nature of samples, as well as the potential risk of exposure to infectious agents or toxic substances, requires particular attention to health and safety standards.

- Personal Protective Equipment (PPE) :
    - This equipment is the first line of defence against the risks of exposure.
    - Gowns, gloves, masks, goggles, headgear and shoe covers are commonly used to protect against splashes, aerosols and particles.
- Handling needles and sharp objects:
    - Correct and safe   handling is essential to prevent injury.
    - Puncture-resistant   containers should be used to safely dispose of sharps after use.
- Disinfection and sterilisation :
    - Surfaces, instruments and equipment must be regularly disinfected to prevent contamination.
    - Autoclaves, which use steam under pressure, are commonly used to sterilise instruments.
- Handling biological samples :

- Aseptic handling techniques must be used to avoid contamination of samples and to protect personnel from infectious agents.
- Biological containment :
  - Forensic laboratories can be equipped with fume hoods and negative pressure rooms to limit the spread of infectious agents.
  - Potentially dangerous samples are often processed in higher-level containment laboratories.
- Waste management :
  - Biological waste must be disposed of safely, generally by incineration or autoclave treatment.
  - Toxic or chemical substances require specialised disposal to avoid contamination of the environment.
- Training and awareness :
  - Regular training of staff in best practice and safety protocols is essential.
  - Emergency procedures, such as handling accidental spills or exposures, must be clearly defined and regularly reviewed.
- Medical follow-up :
  - Forensic professionals must undergo regular medical examinations and may require specific vaccinations to protect against certain diseases.
- Physical security :
  - Given the sensitive nature of the evidence, forensic facilities are often equipped with advanced security systems, such as surveillance cameras, access controls and alarms.

Health and safety precautions in forensic medicine are not only a regulatory necessity, but also an ethical responsibility. They ensure the protection of staff, the accuracy of results and public confidence in the justice system.

Chapter 3:
ROLE AND RESPONSIBILITIES
OF THE FORENSIC NURSE

Autopsy procedures :
assistance and preparation

An autopsy is a complex medical procedure designed to determine the cause of death, assess disease or injury, or study the effects of treatment. Although the forensic pathologist is at the centre of this procedure, the forensic nurse also plays an essential role, particularly in preparation and assistance.

- Preparing the body :
    - On arrival at the morgue, the body is identified and registered.
    - The forensic nurse ensures that the body is placed appropriately on the autopsy table, generally in the dorsal position with the arms extended.
    - Pre-autopsy photographs can be taken to document the initial state of the body and any obvious signs or lesions.
- Assembling the necessary instruments :
    - The nurse prepares a set of surgical instruments, such as scalpels, scissors, forceps, saws and others, ensuring that they are clean, disinfected and ready for use.
- Preparation for taking samples :
    - Tubes, vials and containers are prepared to receive tissue, fluid and organ samples for subsequent analysis.

- Assistance during the external examination :
    - The nurse assists the coroner during the external examination, noting observations, measuring lesions or bruises, and helping to take samples such as fingerprints, hair or fingernails.
- Support when opening the body :
    - The nurse often assists the coroner by holding or lifting parts of the body to facilitate access to internal organs.
    - Fluid samples, such as blood, urine or cerebrospinal fluid, may be taken at this stage.
- Documentation:
    - Throughout the procedure, the forensic nurse records observations, measurements and findings on an autopsy form or in an electronic system.
    - It is essential that this documentation is accurate and detailed, as it can be used as evidence in legal investigations.
- Sample collection and storage :
    - The nurse helps to take tissue samples from various organs for histological examination.
    - These samples are correctly labelled, stored in appropriate solutions and sent to the laboratory for analysis.
- Body closure :
    - Once the autopsy is complete, the nurse assists in the recovery of the body, ensuring that it is treated with respect and dignity.
- Cleaning and disinfection :
    - After the procedure, it is crucial to clean and disinfect the autopsy room, the instruments and any other equipment used. This is essential for safety and hygiene.
- Communication with families :
    - In some cases, the forensic nurse may also play a role in communicating with the families of the

deceased, providing them with information about the autopsy process and responding to their concerns.

Autopsy, although often perceived as a technical procedure, is also profoundly human. The nurse's assistance and preparation ensure not only that the procedure is carried out with rigour and precision, but also with the respect and dignity that each individual deserves after death.

Working with the forensic pathologist

The collaboration between the nurse and the forensic doctor is at the heart of forensic medicine. Together, they form a symbiotic team that ensures that every aspect of the process is carried out with rigour, precision and integrity. This collaboration is based on mutual respect for each other's skills and roles.

- Preliminary assessment :
  - Before the start of any procedure, the nurse and forensic pathologist often consult each other to discuss the information available on the deceased, such as the circumstances of death or medical history.
- Preparation for autopsy :
  - The forensic nurse is generally responsible for preparing the body and gathering the necessary instruments. The forensic pathologist, in turn, may give specific instructions on what to examine in detail or what samples to take.
- Autopsy procedure :
  - During the autopsy, constant communication between the two professionals is essential. The

nurse assists the doctor by providing the necessary instruments, helping with organ handling and taking detailed notes of observations and procedures.

- Consultancy and expertise :
  - In certain complex cases, the nurse can offer a complementary perspective or expertise based on his or her own experience and training. This multidisciplinary collaboration enriches the conclusions and enhances the quality of the investigation.
- Sample management :
  - The nurse is often responsible for collecting, labelling and sending the samples taken for analysis. Clear communication with the forensic pathologist is crucial to ensure that all the necessary samples have been taken and processed correctly.
- Documentation and reports :
  - After the autopsy, the nurse and forensic pathologist often work together to finalise the reports, ensuring that all the information is complete, accurate and consistent. They may also discuss particularly complex or unusual cases to gain mutual perspectives and advice.
- Continuing and advanced training :
  - Forensic medicine is a constantly evolving field. Nurses and forensic scientists often attend training courses, workshops and conferences together to keep abreast of the latest techniques, research and best practice.
- Communication with external parties :
  - In the course of their work, nurses and forensic doctors may be required to collaborate with other professionals, such as investigators, lawyers or family members. Coordinated and unified communication is essential to ensure

that the information shared is clear and consistent.

The collaboration between the forensic nurse and the forensic doctor is fundamental to guaranteeing excellence in forensic medicine. Each brings unique expertise and complementary skills, guaranteeing complete, respectful and accurate handling of each case.

Sample management and traceability

The management and traceability of forensic samples is of paramount importance. Each sample can have crucial forensic significance, and poor management or tracking can compromise not only the scientific integrity of the sample, but also the validity of the evidence in court.

- Sample collection :
  - The time at which a sample is taken is crucial. The nurse must ensure that samples are collected according to standard protocols, using sterilised instruments and avoiding any contamination.
- Labelling and documentation :
  - As soon as a sample is taken, it must be labelled immediately with clear information: name of the deceased, date and time of collection, nature of the sample and identity of the person who took it.
  - This stage is crucial for ensuring the traceability and integrity of the sample throughout its life cycle.
- Storage and preservation :
  - Depending on the nature of the sample, specific storage conditions must be respected, whether refrigeration, freezing or immersion in

a preservative solution. Nurses must know and apply best practice for each type of sample.

- Monitoring system :
  - An effective tracking system is essential. Today, many establishments use electronic systems to ensure real-time traceability of each sample. These systems make it possible to know where the sample is at all times, who has handled it and what analyses have been carried out.
- Transport of samples :
  - If a sample is to be sent to an external laboratory for analysis, strict transport procedures must be followed. These include the use of appropriate packaging, clear labelling and, if necessary, storage conditions during transport.
- Analysis and interpretation :
  - Once the sample is ready for analysis, traceability continues to be essential. Analysis results must be correctly traced back to the original sample and any handling or interpretation must be carefully documented.
- Long-term conservation :
  - In some cases, samples may be kept for long periods, either for legal reasons or for possible future analysis. Long-term storage protocols must ensure that the sample remains intact and uncontaminated.
- Elimination :
  - When a sample is no longer required, it must be disposed of according to specific protocols. This guarantees security, confidentiality and respect for the deceased.

Sample management and traceability are at the heart of the integrity of forensic medicine. By ensuring the careful and rigorous handling of samples, the forensic nurse plays a crucial role in preserving the forensic truth and justice for the deceased and their families.

Chapter 4:
SPECIFIC INTERVENTIONS

Dealing with victims of violence (physical, sexual, etc.)

Interacting with victims of violence is one of the most delicate and crucial responsibilities for forensic nurses. These victims, who are often traumatised and vulnerable, need to be treated with compassion, skill and sensitivity. The nurse's role goes beyond simply collecting evidence; it is a human and empathetic one.

- Welcome and confidence-building :
    - The first step is to provide a safe and welcoming environment for the victim. The nurse must establish a relationship of trust by listening, avoiding judgement and guaranteeing confidentiality.
- Initial assessment :
    - This stage involves determining the medical urgency of the injuries, if any, and ensuring that the victim is physically stable. Urgent medical care may be required before any medico-legal procedure.
- Forensic interview :
    - The nurse takes a detailed history of the events, asking questions in an open and neutral manner. This stage is crucial to understanding what happened and determining what evidence can be gathered.
- Physical examination and collection of evidence :
    - With the victim's consent, the nurse carries out a physical examination. This examination must be carried out with the utmost care and respect, explaining each step to the victim.

Evidence, such as samples or photographs, is collected with precision.

- Preventing after-effects :
  - Depending on the nature of the violence, preventive interventions may be necessary, such as post-exposure prophylaxis for HIV or treatment for STIs. The nurse will also inform the victim of the signs and symptoms to look out for.
- Referral to support services :
  - Victims of violence may need various forms of support, including counselling, support groups and legal aid. The nurse should be aware of the resources available and refer the victim accordingly.
- Documentation and report :
  - The nurse exhaustively documents all observations, victim statements and evidence collected. This documentation can be crucial for subsequent investigations and legal proceedings.
- Follow-up:
  - If necessary, and with the victim's consent, follow-up appointments can be scheduled to monitor medical after-effects or to continue collecting evidence, for example in the case of sexual violence, where certain samples are best collected after a certain period of time.

Caring for victims of violence is an aspect of forensic medicine that requires not only medical expertise, but also a great deal of humanity. The nurse is often the first health professional that the victim meets and, as such, plays a key role in the victim's physical and emotional recovery, while helping to collect evidence that may be essential in bringing about justice.

The nurse dealing with suspicious deaths

When faced with a suspicious death, the forensic nurse plays a central role. Their training and expertise enable them to act as a bridge between the medical and legal worlds, helping to elucidate the circumstances surrounding the death while offering invaluable respect and dignity to the deceased.

- Initial assessment of the body :
    - When the body arrives, the nurse carries out an initial assessment to determine the condition of the deceased, note any obvious signs of trauma or other relevant features, and document any observations.
- Preparation for autopsy :
    - The nurse prepares the body for the post-mortem examination. This may include cleaning the body, taking preliminary photographs, and setting up the instruments needed for the autopsy.
- Assistance at autopsy :
    - During the autopsy, the nurse works closely with the forensic pathologist, providing instruments, helping to collect samples and documenting observations.
- Evidence gathering :
    - In the context of a suspicious death, every detail can be crucial. The nurse ensures that all samples are correctly taken, preserved and documented, guaranteeing their integrity for any subsequent analyses or presentations in court.
- Communication with investigators :
    - The nurse may be required to communicate directly with the police, providing relevant

medical details that may help the investigation into the cause of death.
- Managing emotions and stress :
  - Faced with a suspicious death, nurses can be confronted with emotionally challenging scenes. It is essential that they have the tools and support they need to manage the stress and emotional impact of their work.
- Continuing education and training :
  - As forensic techniques and investigation methods are constantly evolving, nurses need to keep abreast of the latest developments, by attending regular training courses and keeping up to date with best practice.
- Communication with families :
  - In some cases, nurses may be asked to provide information to bereaved families, while respecting confidentiality limits and established protocols.

Suspicious death brings with it its share of mystery, pain and uncertainty. For the forensic nurse, it means navigating this complex landscape with skill, compassion and integrity, playing an essential role in the quest for truth and justice while honouring the dignity of those who have died.

Specific aspects of care children and vulnerable people

Forensic nurses dealing with children or vulnerable people, whether elderly, disabled or other fragile populations, must show particular care, empathy and skill. These individuals are often more likely to suffer harm, less able to report it and require care tailored to their specific needs.

- Adapted communication :
  - It is essential to establish a method of communication that takes account of the person's cognitive and emotional abilities. With children, this may mean using simplified language or visual aids. For people with disabilities, it may mean using alternative methods of communication.
- Reassuring atmosphere:
  - The forensic environment can be intimidating. Creating a safe environment, perhaps with toys for children or familiar objects for the elderly, can help reduce anxiety.
- Appropriate physical examination :
  - Examining a child or vulnerable person may require specific techniques or extra patience. It is crucial to ensure that the individual feels safe and understood.
- Recognising signs of trauma :
  - Children and vulnerable people may show signs of trauma in different ways. Nurses must be trained to recognise these subtle and appropriate signs.
- Working with specialist departments:
  - Often, other professionals, such as social workers, psychologists or advocates, may be involved. Effective collaboration is essential to ensure the well-being of the individual.
- Accurate documentation :
  - When dealing with vulnerable populations, accurate documentation is crucial. This can include details of how the information was gathered, any witnesses present and the measures taken to ensure the person's comfort.
- Educating families and carers:
  - Families and carers play an essential role in supporting vulnerable people. Informing and

educating them about what to expect, the signs of trauma and the resources available is vital.

- Respect and dignity :
  - Beyond all the techniques and skills, it is fundamental to treat each individual, whatever their ability or age, with the utmost respect and dignity.

Caring for children and vulnerable people in forensic medicine is both a rewarding and complex challenge. Nurses must constantly balance the need to obtain accurate forensic information with the need to provide compassionate and appropriate care to individuals who are often in great distress.

Chapter 5:
FORENSIC TECHNIQUES

Withdrawals
and toxicological analyses

In forensic medicine, toxicological samples and analyses play a crucial role. They can help determine the cause of death, establish the presence of substances in the system of a victim or suspect, or provide evidence in criminal cases. Nurses, in collaboration with other health professionals, are often involved in this delicate process.

- Background to toxicological analyses :
    - Toxicological samples may be requested for a variety of reasons, such as suspected poisoning, overdose, driving under the influence or exposure to toxic agents.
- Types of samples :
    - **Blood**: the most common sample taken to determine the presence and concentration of substances.
    - **Urine**: useful for detecting the presence of drugs or their metabolites.
    - **Hair**: may indicate long-term exposure or drug use over a prolonged period.
    - **Saliva: increasingly** used for rapid screening tests.
    - **Organic tissue: in the** case of autopsies, to search for specific toxins or metabolites.
- Sampling protocol :
    - Hygiene is essential to avoid contamination. Nurses must use sterile gloves and ensure that containers are properly sealed and labelled.

- Traceability is essential. Each sample must be correctly labelled with details such as name, date, time and place of sampling.
- Transport and storage :
  - Samples must be kept at the right temperature and transported quickly to the laboratory for analysis. Compliance with the protocols ensures the integrity of the sample.
- Interpretation of results :
  - The presence of a substance does not necessarily mean that it is the cause of a symptom or death. Understanding therapeutic, toxic and lethal levels is crucial. Nurses must also be aware of possible interactions between different drugs or substances.
- Ethics and confidentiality :
  - As with all medical procedures, ethics must be respected. Permission must be obtained (except in certain legal circumstances) and the confidentiality of results maintained.
- Communication with other professionals :
  - The nurse may need to communicate the results to forensic scientists, investigators or other health professionals. A clear understanding of the context and implications of the results is essential.

Toxicological samples and analyses are powerful tools in the world of forensic medicine. They can reveal hidden truths, shed light on medical mysteries or provide invaluable evidence in legal proceedings. For the nurse, competence, precision and integrity are fundamental to this process.

The importance of the chain of custody for evidence

The chain of custody is an essential element in the forensic field. It guarantees the integrity, traceability and credibility of the evidence collected, ensuring that it can be used with confidence in legal proceedings.

- Definition of the chain of custody :
  - The chain of custody is a process that documents the possession, transfer, handling and storage of evidence, from the time it is collected until it is presented in court or disposed of.
- Ensuring the integrity of evidence :
  - For evidence to be admissible in court, it must be shown that it has not been altered, contaminated or falsified in any way. A well-documented chain of custody is a guarantee that the evidence has been handled with the utmost care.
- Avoiding legal controversy:
  - A broken or poorly documented chain of custody can lead to the validity of evidence being called into question. This can lead to the exclusion of evidence from a trial or, in some cases, the quashing of a conviction.
- Responsibility and role of the nurse :
  - Nurses play a key role in maintaining the chain of custody, particularly when collecting biological samples or other medical evidence. Accurate documentation, secure storage and correct handover of samples are crucial.
- Standardised protocols :
  - To ensure a uniform and reliable chain of custody, standardised protocols must be in place. This includes the use of sealed

packaging, identification labels and appropriate documentation forms.
- Traceability :
  - Every time evidence is transferred from one person to another or handled, this must be duly recorded. This traceability ensures that the complete history of the handling of a piece of evidence can be traced.
- Training and awareness :
  - Professionals involved in the collection, processing or management of evidence must be properly trained in the importance of the chain of custody. This ensures that errors are minimised and protocols are followed.
- Consequences of a broken chain of custody :
  - Beyond the legal implications, a broken chain of custody can lead to a loss of confidence in the legal system, misidentification and, in some cases, injustice for those involved.

The chain of custody of evidence is more than just an administrative process: it is the foundation of judicial integrity. For the forensic nurse, understanding and respecting this chain is not only a professional responsibility but also an ethical duty towards justice and the truth.

Technological advances : DNA, imaging, etc.

Forensic science, like many other medical fields, has been profoundly transformed by technological advances. These innovations have increased the accuracy, efficiency and reliability of analyses, offering unprecedented opportunities to solve complex legal cases and better understand the circumstances surrounding a death or trauma.

- DNA analysis :
    - **Introduction and impact**: DNA identification has revolutionised crime solving. It enables precise identification from tiny biological samples, making it possible to solve unsolved cases dating back decades.
    - **Advanced techniques**: Methods such as next-generation sequencing make it possible to analyse degraded or mixed DNA samples, increasing the chances of obtaining a usable genetic profile.
    - **Limits and ethics**: While DNA is a powerful tool, it also raises ethical questions about privacy, data storage and human rights.
- Medical imaging in forensic medicine :
    - **Computed tomography (CT)**: Provides a detailed 3D image of the internal organs, often used to determine the cause of death without the need for an invasive autopsy.
    - **Magnetic Resonance Imaging (MRI)**: Used to visualise soft tissues, it can help identify trauma or specific pathologies.
    - **Radiography**: Although this is an older technique, it is still invaluable for visualising fractures, foreign objects or bone lesions.
- Digital identification technologies :
    - **Facial recognition**: Although controversial, this technology can help identify victims or suspects from CCTV footage or photos.
    - **Digitised fingerprints**: The use of high-resolution scanners means that fingerprints can be analysed quickly and accurately, facilitating database matches.
- Modern toxicology :
    - With the development of mass spectrometry and other advanced techniques, laboratories can now detect extremely low concentrations

of substances, including synthetic drugs that have recently appeared on the market.

- Digital applications and software :
  - Modelling software can help to reconstruct crime scenes or bullet trajectories. In addition, centralised databases enable information to be shared and analysed rapidly, speeding up investigations.
- 3D printing in forensic medicine:
  - 3D printers can be used to create replicas of bones, weapons or other pieces of evidence, making them easier to visualise and analyse.
- Challenges and precautions :
  - Despite their advantages, these technologies are not infallible. Errors, whether due to technical or human problems or contamination, can have serious legal consequences. In addition, there are ethical and legal issues surrounding privacy, data retention and consent.

Technological advances in forensic medicine offer exciting opportunities for professionals in the field, including nurses. However, with these opportunities come responsibilities, requiring ongoing training, ethical awareness and rigorous adherence to standardised protocols.

Chapter 6:
PSYCHOLOGICAL AND ETHICAL ASPECTS

Bereaved families Support

At the heart of forensic medicine, beyond the technical procedures, analyses and reports, is the human element. The forensic nurse is often one of the first health professionals to interact with bereaved families. This support, which combines sensitivity, professionalism and ethics, is essential to help loved ones through this painful period.

- Understanding the grieving process :
    - Grief is a natural response to loss, but it has no fixed chronology or uniform manifestation. Each person, each family, goes through grief in its own way.
- The first meeting :
    - The first moments of contact with a bereaved family are crucial. The approach must be one of empathy, respect and sincerity. Tone of voice, choice of words and body language all play an essential role in creating a safe and respectful space.
- Clear and transparent communication:
    - Families are looking for answers. Although there may be information that cannot or should not be shared immediately, it is important to be as transparent and direct as possible, while remaining sensitive.
- Respecting cultural and religious rituals :
    - Every culture and religion has its own rites and customs surrounding death. It is essential to be aware of them, to respect them and to

incorporate them as far as possible into interactions and procedures.
- Referral to specialist resources :
    - Nurses alone cannot meet all the needs of a bereaved family. It is therefore crucial to know which specialist organisations and professionals (psychologists, bereavement counsellors, support groups) to refer families to.
- Managing personal emotions :
    - Supporting bereaved families is emotionally demanding. Nurses must also take care of themselves, seek support if necessary and recognise when they need to step back.
- Maintaining confidentiality :
    - Discretion is fundamental. Details of the circumstances surrounding a death or court case must remain confidential, unless it is legally or ethically necessary to share them.
- The rest of the process :
    - Even after the first meeting, the support can continue. Whether it's to share test results, answer questions later or simply offer ongoing support, the nurse remains a pillar for the family.

Supporting bereaved families is an often underestimated aspect of forensic medicine. However, for many families, the nurse can be a beacon in the storm, a reassuring and professional presence, guiding loved ones through one of the most difficult periods of their lives.

Stress management and preserving mental health

The profession of forensic nursing involves unique emotional, psychological and sometimes even physical challenges. Faced regularly with death, suffering and the distress of families, these professionals are subject to considerable stress. It is imperative that they have the tools and resources they need to manage this stress and preserve their mental health.

- Recognising the signs :
    - The first symptoms of stress or burnout can be subtle: irritability, fatigue, insomnia, feelings of isolation or anxiety. Recognising these signs is the first step in dealing with them.
- Establishing borders :
    - While compassion and empathy are essential in this profession, it is also important to know how to set limits. This ensures a balance between professional and personal life, avoiding emotional overload.
- Developing relaxation techniques :
    - Whether it's meditation, yoga, deep breathing or any other technique, these methods can help you refocus, reduce anxiety and manage everyday stress.
- Seeking professional support :
    - There is no shame in asking for help. Therapy or counselling can offer strategies for managing stress, dealing with trauma and preventing burnout.
- Establish a support network :
    - Colleagues, friends, family or specialist support groups can provide a listening ear, share experiences and offer different perspectives.

- Taking care of yourself physically:
    - A balanced diet, regular exercise and sufficient sleep are essential for managing stress and maintaining sound mental health.
- Ritualising the end of the day:
    - It can be useful to have a ritual to mark the end of the working day and the transition to personal life, be it a walk, a moment of reading or any other relaxing activity.
- Further training and supervision :
    - Taking part in workshops or training courses on stress management or mental health can be beneficial. Supervision sessions also provide a safe space to discuss professional challenges.
- Taking breaks:
    - If possible, take time out during the day to rest. What's more, taking a holiday or time off can help you recharge your batteries and prevent exhaustion.
- Recognising your limits:
    - It's crucial to admit when you're overwhelmed and talk to a supervisor or colleague. Sometimes a simple adjustment of responsibilities can make all the difference.

Managing stress and maintaining mental health are not signs of weakness, but of strength. For a forensic nurse, this guarantees not only their own health and well-being, but also the quality of care and support they offer to others.

Ethical dilemmas
in forensic medicine

In forensic medicine, science and justice intersect, giving rise to a series of unique ethical dilemmas. As the pivot between these two worlds, nurses regularly find themselves confronted with complex ethical issues. It is essential to approach them with reflection, integrity and respect.

- Conflict between justice and care:
  - Nurses are first and foremost trained to provide care. But in forensic medicine, the search for the judicial truth can sometimes come into conflict with the need for care. How can these two responsibilities be reconciled?
- Confidentiality versus disclosure :
  - Protecting medical information is a pillar of medical ethics. However, in forensic medicine, certain elements may be required by the courts. When and how should this information be disclosed, and to what extent?
- Consent in a judicial context :
  - Legal procedures may require examinations or samples to be taken. How can we ensure that the patient or family gives informed consent, especially when they are in shock or in mourning?
- Treatment of prisoners and human rights :
  - When carrying out medical examinations on detainees or suspects, how can nurses guarantee ethical treatment, especially in contexts where human rights could be compromised?
- Impartiality and bias :
  - Nurses must remain neutral, but unconscious prejudices can influence observations and decisions. How can constant impartiality be guaranteed?
- Interactions with the family :
  - In autopsy or suspicious death situations, families can be distressed and even angry. How do you navigate between the emotional

needs of loved ones and the demands of the legal process?
- Autopsy decision against religious or cultural will :
  - Some cultures and religions have reservations about or prohibitions on autopsies. How can these beliefs be respected while ensuring that legal and medical requirements are met?
- Emerging technologies and consent :
  - With advances in technologies such as genomic sequencing, new ethical issues are emerging. How can we ensure that patients understand the implications of these tests?
- Training and learning on bodies :
  - The use of bodies for training or research is crucial, but it also raises ethical questions. How can we guarantee respect for the deceased and their families?
- Handling failure or error :
  - In forensic medicine, an error can have major legal consequences. How do you manage these situations, take responsibility and ensure that justice is done?

Ethical dilemmas in forensic medicine require deep reflection, respect for the rights of individuals and a constant commitment to integrity. For the nurse, they represent both a challenge and an opportunity to strengthen public confidence in the judicial and medical system.

Chapter 7:
CASE STUDIES AND FEEDBACK

Analysis of real cases: lessons learned

The analysis of real-life forensic cases provides a valuable learning opportunity. Not only does it allow us to understand the nuances of real-life situations, but it also provides essential lessons for improving practice. Although each case is unique, they often offer common lessons.

- **The case of inadequate sampling :**
- During an autopsy, inappropriate sampling compromised the toxicological results, hampering the judicial process.
    - **Lesson**: Rigour and precision in sample collection are crucial. Ongoing training and updating of skills guarantee the reliability of procedures.
- **Death due to a rare disease:**
- A woman died suddenly, and the initial autopsy did not reveal the cause. However, a careful review of the family history revealed a rare hereditary heart disease.
    - **Lesson**: The importance of a complete medical history and analysis of family history. Non-medical information can be just as vital as clinical data.
- **Mistaken identification of the body :**
- Two victims of a road accident have been incorrectly identified, causing immense distress to their families.
    - **Lesson**: Identification procedures must be meticulous and multi-faceted, incorporating methods such as dental impressions, DNA and visual identification by relatives.

- **The distress of an uninformed family :**
- An autopsy was carried out without fully informing the family of the details, causing a breach of trust.
    - **Lesson**: Transparent and empathetic communication with families is essential. Respect for their feelings and rights is paramount.
- **An error of judgement when faced with signs of violence:**
- One deceased individual had slight bruising, initially dismissed as benign. Further investigation revealed a violent cause.
    - **Lesson**: Caution must be exercised, even in the face of subtle signs. Every mark or lesion must be carefully examined and documented.
- **Lack of interdisciplinary collaboration :**
- In a complex case involving possible poisoning, a lack of communication between the experts delayed resolution.
    - **Lesson**: Forensic medicine is a collaborative effort. Open communication between nurses, forensic scientists, toxicologists and other specialists is crucial.
- **Neglect of psychological follow-up :**
- After being exposed to a series of traumatic incidents, a nurse developed post-traumatic stress disorder.
    - **Lesson**: The mental health of forensic professionals is paramount. Psychological support must be integrated into the professional framework.

Analysis of these cases highlights the complexity and responsibility inherent in forensic medicine. By learning from each situation, professionals can continually refine their skills, ensuring the highest quality of service for justice, the deceased and their families.

Mistakes to avoid

Forensic medicine, as the bridge between medicine and justice, is an area where mistakes can have profound consequences, not only for the families of the deceased, but also for legal proceedings. Here is a list of common mistakes to avoid, together with recommendations to ensure ethical and professional practice.

- Neglect of documentation :
    - All information, no matter how insignificant, must be accurately recorded.
    - Recommendation: Use a checklist to ensure that all steps are documented.
- Failure to comply with hygiene protocols :
    - Even under pressure, health protocols must be respected.
    - Recommendation: Regularly review and update training on good hygiene practices.
- Communicating results prematurely:
    - Providing information before all the analyses have been completed can be misleading.
    - Recommendation: Ensure that all results are finalised and reviewed before communicating them.
- Ignoring or minimising the importance of the chain of custody of evidence :
    - Any interruption may call into question the validity of the samples.
    - Recommendation: Strictly follow procedures and document every step in the chain.
- Rely exclusively on personal experience rather than established protocols:
    - Experience is valuable, but it does not replace standard procedures.
    - Recommendation: Encourage a culture of respect for protocols while valuing experience.

- Neglecting the emotional well-being of loved ones:
  - Families are often in mourning and need empathetic communication.
  - Recommendation: Offer compassionate communication training to your team.
- Underestimating the emotional impact on yourself:
  - Ignoring your own well-being can lead to burnout.
  - Recommendation: Incorporate regular wellbeing assessments and offer psychological support.
- Lack of updates and ongoing training:
  - Forensic medicine is constantly evolving, particularly with technological advances.
  - Recommendation: Encourage ongoing training to keep up to date.
- Drawing hasty conclusions without concrete evidence:
  - A hasty conclusion can distort the truth.
  - Recommendation: Approach each case with an open, fact-based mentality.
- Neglecting interdisciplinary collaboration :
  - Forensic medicine requires the expertise of various professionals.
  - Recommendation: Facilitate and encourage collaboration between the various experts.
- Not recognising your own limits:
  - No one is infallible; it's crucial to know when to ask for help or a second opinion.
  - Recommendation: Cultivate a culture of humility and collaboration within the team.

By avoiding these errors, the forensic nurse can guarantee respectful, professional practice in the service of justice and the truth.

Testimonials from nurses forensic medicine experts

Note: The following testimonials are fictitious, but are intended to illustrate the diversity and depth of experience of forensic nurses.

Camille, 10 years' experience :
"For me, forensic science is much more than just a job; it's a vocation. Each case reminds me of the importance of our role - not only in the search for the truth, but also in supporting bereaved families. Once, after a particularly delicate autopsy, I spent an hour with the family, answering their questions and helping them to find some peace. It's these moments that give deep meaning to my job."

Khaled, 15 years' experience :
"I remember one case where the initial clues seemed clear, but something told me we might have missed something. After re-running the tests and seeking the advice of a colleague, we discovered a rare genetic anomaly. Not only did this shed light on the cause of death, it also enabled the family to get tested and take preventive measures. Rigour and perseverance are essential in this profession."

Elena, 7 years' experience :
"What many people don't realise is the emotional weight we carry. Yes, we are trained to do this, but each case, each body has a history, a family. It's a constant challenge to navigate between our professional duty and our humanity. Fortunately, I have an incredible team around me, and we support each other through the most difficult days."

Raj, 20 years' experience:
"With advances in technology, our field has evolved enormously. What used to be a procedure lasting several

days can now be done in a few hours thanks to technology. However, the most rewarding aspect for me remains the collaboration with my colleagues. Together, we combine our knowledge and expertise to solve the most complex puzzles."

Léa, 5 years' experience :
"I entered forensic medicine after working in intensive care. The transition was a shock, but I quickly understood the importance of our role. Every victim deserves justice and dignity, and that's what we strive to provide, day in, day out. And even though some days are harder than others, I know I'm contributing to something much bigger than myself."

These fictional accounts seek to highlight the challenges, rewards and passion that drive forensic nurses. Each case has its own mysteries to solve, families to comfort, and truths to uncover.

Chapter 8:
THE RELATIONSHIP
CROSS-INDUSTRY

Working with the police and investigators

The interaction between medical staff and the police is an essential aspect of forensic medicine. When properly conducted, this collaboration not only sheds light on the circumstances of a death or assault, but also brings justice to the victim and answers to his or her relatives. As a key member of the forensic team, the nurse plays a pivotal role in this alliance.

1. Interprofessional communication :
One of the key skills for a forensic nurse is the ability to communicate effectively with police and investigators. This means conveying complex medical information in a way that is understandable to those without a medical background, while ensuring that crucial details are not lost.

2. Evidence gathering :
In many cases, the nurse may be the first medical professional to examine a live victim, for example in cases of sexual violence. It is therefore essential that they know how to collect, preserve and document physical evidence that could be used in an investigation or trial.

3. Crime scenes :
Sometimes the nurse is called to a crime scene to help assess and preserve medical evidence. In these situations, it is crucial to understand the investigation protocols so as not to compromise the evidence.

4. Expert testimony :
A specialist nurse may be called to testify in court as an expert, sharing their observations and medical findings to

help the jury or judge understand the medical elements of a case.

5. Further training :
Investigators and police may not be familiar with the latest medical techniques or discoveries. Nurses can organise or take part in seminars and training courses for law enforcement officers, ensuring a mutual and up-to-date understanding of procedures and knowledge.

6. Mutual respect and trust :
The relationship between the nurse and the investigators is based on trust. It is essential that each party understands and respects the role and expertise of the other to ensure a fruitful collaboration.

7. Managing emotions :
Crime scenes and forensic cases can be emotionally charged. Nurses, like investigators, need to know how to manage their emotions in order to remain objective and professional.

The collaboration between the forensic nurse, the police and the investigators is crucial to the search for the truth. Together, they form a close-knit team whose aim is to bring justice and clarity to the darkest and most complex cases.

Working with psychologists, psychiatrists and social workers

Forensic medicine, with its complex and often emotional nuances, requires a collaborative approach. While nurses, forensic doctors and the police play crucial roles, the support of psychologists, psychiatrists and social workers is equally vital to ensure holistic care for all those involved, whether victims, their families or even medical staff.

1. Support for victims :
   - **Psychosocial approach**: After a trauma, a victim may need help to deal with the emotional shock. Social workers can provide immediate support, draw up an intervention plan and refer the victim to appropriate services.
   - **Psychiatric assessment**: In some cases, the victim may present symptoms that require psychiatric assessment, whether for post-traumatic stress disorder, suicidal tendencies or other conditions.
   - **Ongoing therapy**: A psychologist or psychiatrist can provide long-term therapy to help the victim overcome the trauma.
2. Support for families :
   - **Bereavement support**: Social workers can guide families through the early stages of bereavement, helping them to understand and manage their emotions.
   - **Referral to support groups**: Families can benefit from support groups where they can share their experiences and feel less isolated.
   - **Conflict intervention**: Tensions can arise in families following a death or trauma. A psychologist or social worker can intervene to ease these tensions.
3. Support for medical staff :
   - **Stress management**: Faced with emotionally charged situations, medical staff may feel stressed, tired or even burnt out. Regular sessions with a psychologist or stress management workshops can help.
   - **Debriefing after difficult cases**: After a particularly troubling case, a debriefing session with a psychologist can help staff to process their emotions and find strategies for moving forward.
   - **Psychiatric consultations**: In extreme situations, some professionals may require psychiatric

assessment and follow-up to ensure their mental well-being.

4. Interprofessional collaboration and training :

- **Joint training**: Training sessions where nurses, forensic doctors, social workers, psychologists and psychiatrists learn together can strengthen collaboration and ensure a better understanding of each other's roles.
- **Multidisciplinary case studies**: Regularly discussing cases from different professional angles can enrich the overall care of victims and their families.

In forensic medicine, interdisciplinary collaboration is essential to ensure comprehensive and respectful care. Each professional brings a unique expertise which, when combined, provides a solid network of support and intervention for all concerned.

Interaction with lawyers and the judicial system

At the crossroads between medicine and the law, the forensic nurse plays an essential role, which inevitably involves interaction with the legal world. This collaboration ensures that medical evidence is used correctly in legal proceedings and that justice is done fairly.

1. Preparing testimonials :

- **Understanding legal expectations**: Nurses must be prepared to explain their findings in a way that is understandable to a legal audience, while remaining medically accurate.
- **Testimonial simulation**: Working with lawyers to practise giving evidence can help prepare you for the pressure of the courtroom.

2. The role of expert witness :
- **Presentation of evidence**: The nurse may be required to present medical evidence, such as autopsy reports or samples, and explain its relevance.
- **Answering questions**: Communication skills are essential for answering questions from defence and prosecution lawyers, often in tense situations.

3. Navigating the legal system :
- **Understanding the judicial process**: It is crucial to understand how the system works, from the first hearings to the trial, so that you can better interact with the lawyers and the court.
- **Compliance with legal procedures**: Nurses must be familiar with and comply with the protocols for presenting evidence, preserving samples and giving evidence.

4. Confidentiality and ethics :
- **Protection of sensitive information**: Nurses must ensure that all medical information remains confidential, except when it is required for legal proceedings.
- **Professional integrity**: It is essential to be honest and transparent, avoiding any bias or partiality in the presentation of evidence or testimony.

5. Working with lawyers :
- **Joint preparation**: Prior discussions with the lawyers help to clarify the nurse's role in the trial and anticipate any questions.
- **Ongoing training**: Organise training sessions with lawyers to better understand the legal implications of medical evidence and testimony.

6. Pressure management :
- **Emotional support**: Interactions with the legal system can be stressful. Finding ways to manage this stress, such as meditation or consulting mental health professionals, can be beneficial.

- **Keep up to date**: Laws and procedures change. Ongoing training is essential to stay informed and effective in this interdisciplinary role.

Interaction with lawyers and the justice system is a crucial dimension of the forensic nurse's work. By skilfully navigating this interface, the nurse helps to ensure that medicine and justice work together seamlessly, for the benefit of society as a whole.

Chapter 9:
MEDICO-LEGAL ASPECTS
IN SPECIFIC CONTEXTS

Forensic medicine in context
natural disasters
or terrorist acts

In exceptional situations, such as natural disasters or acts of terrorism, forensic medicine is faced with immense challenges that are often unpredictable and urgent. These tragic events require seamless coordination between different professional sectors to identify victims, provide support to their families and contribute to investigations.

1. Managing the drama scene :
   - **Securing the site**: After an act of terrorism or a natural disaster, it is vital to secure the area before any forensic procedures are undertaken.
   - **Initial sorting**: With a high number of victims, it is crucial to sort the bodies quickly, take samples and document the scene.
2. Victim identification :
   - **Logistical challenges**: Major disasters can result in a large number of deaths, requiring meticulous organisation to manage identification.
   - **Use of technology**: DNA, dental prints and other methods are used to accurately identify victims when visual identification is not possible.
3. Inter-agency collaboration :
   - **Constant communication**: In these situations, forensic nurses need to work closely with other professionals, including the police, fire brigade, emergency services and government agencies.

- **Coordination centres**: Specific centres can be set up to manage the crisis, where information is centralised and disseminated efficiently.

4. Support for the families of the victims :
- **Information centres**: Dedicated places can be set up to inform families about the identification process and updates concerning their loved ones.
- **Psychological support**: Given the emotional shock, psychological support must be put in place quickly for bereaved families.

5. Collection and preservation of evidence :
- **Investigations**: In the case of terrorist acts, medical evidence can be essential to the criminal investigation.
- **Unique challenges**: Natural disasters can compromise the conservation of samples due to environmental conditions, requiring rapid adaptations.

6. Preparation and training :
- **Disaster simulations**: Training based on disaster scenarios can help forensic nurses prepare for real-life interventions.
- **International collaboration**: In some cases, particularly for large-scale events, international collaboration may be necessary, involving specialist teams from other countries.

7. Managing work-related stress :
- **Post-traumatic debriefing**: Given the seriousness and scale of these events, professionals may need psychological support to deal with post-traumatic stress.
- **Team rotation**: To avoid burnout, it may be necessary to rotate teams regularly in the field.

Intervening in forensic medicine in the context of natural disasters or acts of terrorism requires not only medical expertise, but also the ability to act quickly, collaborate on a large scale and demonstrate great emotional resilience.

These interventions are essential to bring justice to victims, support their families and contribute to the overall investigation.

The role of the forensic nurse in contexts of war or conflict

Wars and armed conflicts present unique challenges for forensic medicine. In these contexts, the forensic nurse plays an essential role in guaranteeing respect for human rights, documenting war crimes and caring for victims. Intervention sites can be unpredictable, with situations that can change rapidly.

1. Identifying victims of conflict :
   - **Mass casualties**: Conflicts can generate a large number of victims in a short space of time, requiring rapid and systematic identification efforts.
   - **Exhumations**: In some cases, forensic nurses may have to exhume mass graves or mass graves to identify bodies.
2. Documentation of war crimes :
   - **Evidence gathering**: Forensic nurses are often at the forefront of documenting evidence of torture, genocide or other crimes against humanity.
   - **Collaboration with international courts**: Evidence gathered may be used before international courts, such as the International Criminal Court.
3. Management of war injuries :
   - **Treatment of specific injuries**: Armed conflicts can result in specific types of injury, such as those caused by landmines or chemical weapons.
   - **Infection prevention** : In conflict zones, access to medical care may be limited, making the prevention of secondary infections crucial.

4. Working together in hostile zones :
- **Working with NGOs and international bodies**: In war zones, collaboration with organisations such as the Red Cross or Médecins Sans Frontières is essential.
- **Personal safety**: The safety of forensic nurses may be at risk. They must therefore be trained in safety protocols for conflict zones.

5. Psychological support for victims :
- **Multiple trauma**: War victims may have suffered both physical and psychological trauma. The treatment of these traumas is therefore multidimensional.
- **Referrals and liaison** : Forensic nurses must be able to refer victims to appropriate specialists, such as psychologists or social workers.

6. Specific training :
- **Preparing for war**: Training for forensic nurses to work in conflict zones needs to be stepped up, covering medical, ethical and security aspects.
- **Regular updates**: As combat methods and weaponry evolve, ongoing training is crucial.

7. Ethics and neutrality :
- **Professional neutrality**: In wartime contexts, neutrality is essential to guarantee access to victims and respect by all parties to the conflict.
- **Respect for international humanitarian law**: Forensic nurses must be well informed about the conventions and treaties that protect victims and medical personnel in wartime.

In war zones, forensic nurses play a vital role despite a particularly complex and dangerous working environment. Their mission goes beyond the simple application of medical skills, as it involves a deep understanding of the human and legal issues at stake. These professionals thus become major players in documenting the consequences of conflicts, defending human rights and seeking justice for victims.

Unsolved disappearances

Unsolved disappearances are an enigma for investigators, families and the community. These cases, steeped in mystery and uncertainty, require meticulous attention and extensive expertise. For the forensic nurse, these disappearances present particular challenges, as they may involve the analysis of human remains discovered long after the initial disappearance.

1. The late discovery of human remains :
   - **Deterioration and decomposition**: Bodies found long after a disappearance may be badly decomposed or skeletal, making identification difficult.
   - **Impact of natural elements**: Factors such as temperature, humidity and fauna can alter the conservation of bodies and influence analyses.
2. Identification of remains :
   - **Use of DNA**: In cases where the remains are severely degraded, DNA may be the only reliable means of identification.
   - **Dental and bone analysis**: These methods can help determine the age, sex and other characteristics of the missing person.
3. Collaboration with other experts :
   - **Anthropologists and forensic odontologists**: These specialists can provide valuable expertise in the analysis of human remains.
   - **Database professionals**: Information on missing persons can be cross-referenced with national or international databases to facilitate identification.

4. Support for families :
- **Delicate communication**: Informing a family of the potential discovery of a loved one requires compassion and tact.
- **Psychological help**: Families may need psychological support when faced with confirmation of the death of a loved one.

5. Investigation into the circumstances of the disappearance :
- **Searching for clues to the cause of death**: The forensic nurse analyses the remains for signs of trauma or other clues to the cause of death.
- **Working with the investigators**: Smooth communication with the investigators is essential to help solve the mystery of the disappearance.

6. Specific training and preparation :
- **Regular updates**: The development of identification techniques requires ongoing training for forensic nurses.
- **Stress management**: Dealing with unsolved disappearances can be emotionally taxing, requiring stress management strategies.

7. Role in prevention and education :
- **Raising public awareness**: The forensic nurse can help to raise public awareness of the importance of promptly reporting disappearances.
- **Training the police**: Educating the police on how to deal with the critical first few hours of a disappearance can be crucial.

Unsolved disappearances are an ordeal for everyone involved. Forensic nurses play a central role in the effort to provide answers to families in search of the truth. Although each case is unique, the expertise, compassion and determination of these professionals remain constant in their quest to unravel the darkest mysteries.

Chapter 10:
CULTURAL ISSUES
AND SOCIETAL ISSUES IN FORENSIC
MEDICINE

Respect for funeral rites
and cultural beliefs

As well as devoting themselves to their scientific mission, forensic nurses must also take account of the values, beliefs and traditions of bereaved families. Recognising and respecting funeral rites and cultural beliefs are essential to guaranteeing the dignity of the deceased and ensuring harmonious collaboration with families and communities.

1. Understanding different funeral traditions :
    • **Variety of rites**: Funeral traditions vary considerably between cultures, religions and regions of the world.
    • **Implications for autopsy**: Certain rites require rapid burial or prohibit certain interventions on the body.
2. Working with families :
    • **Respectful communication**: Establishing an open dialogue with families helps us to better understand their expectations and specific needs.
    • **Participation in rituals**: In certain contexts, the presence of medical professionals may be required or appreciated during ceremonies.
3. Adapting protocols :
    • **Respecting deadlines**: Some cultures require burial within hours of death.
    • **Handling the body**: The approach must be respectful of beliefs, for example by avoiding certain incisions or using specific sheets.

4. Cultural training for forensic personnel :
- **Awareness of different beliefs**: Ongoing training enables forensic nurses to remain informed and respectful of different traditions.
- **Practical scenarios**: Case studies can help staff to navigate culturally sensitive situations.

5. Working with community leaders :
- **Mediation**: Religious or community leaders can act as mediators between forensic personnel and families.
- **Education**: These leaders can also help to educate the community about the importance of forensic medicine, while ensuring that rites are respected.

6. Respect for diversity within the forensic team :
- **Multicultural teams**: Having a diverse team can enrich understanding and respect for different beliefs.
- **Sharing experiences**: Team members can share their knowledge and perspectives on different funeral traditions.

7. Recognition of potential tensions :
- **Conflicts between medical protocols and beliefs**: In some cases, medico-legal requirements may conflict with funeral traditions. Navigating these situations requires diplomacy and creativity.
- **Emotional support**: Providing emotional support to bereaved families is essential, especially when cultural tensions arise.

Respecting funeral rites and cultural beliefs is more than just a courtesy; it is an ethical imperative for forensic nurses. By taking traditions into account and working closely with families and communities, these professionals can ensure the dignity of the deceased and facilitate the grieving process, while fulfilling their crucial mission within forensic medicine.

Legal differences
and procedures between countries

Forensic medicine, although based on universal scientific principles, is profoundly influenced by the legal, cultural and social contexts of each country. For the forensic nurse, understanding these differences is essential, whether to work abroad, collaborate with international colleagues or simply to keep abreast of global best practice.

1. Judicial systems :
   - **Common Law vs. Civil Law**: The distinction between these two major legal systems influences the way forensic medicine is practised, particularly in terms of evidence and testimony.
   - **Expert roles**: In some countries, the forensic nurse may be called upon to give expert evidence in court, while in others this role is assigned exclusively to the forensic doctor.
2. Autopsy procedures :
   - **Indications for autopsy**: Some countries may require autopsies in specific circumstances, such as sudden or unexplained deaths, while others give doctors more latitude.
   - **Family consent**: The need to obtain the consent of relatives varies from one jurisdiction to another, influenced by cultural and religious considerations.
3. Respect for human rights :
   - **Treatment of prisoners**: The way in which deceased prisoners are treated medico-legally can vary, especially in countries where human rights are less respected.
   - **Identifying victims of conflict**: Some countries have set up special procedures to identify victims of war or genocide.

4. Training and qualifications :

- **Academic requirements**: The qualifications needed to become a forensic nurse can vary considerably from one country to another.
- **Professional accreditation**: Some countries have professional organisations that accredit or certify forensic nurses, while others rely on academic institutions.

5. International collaboration :

- **Cross-border organisations**: Organisations such as INTERPOL facilitate collaboration in forensic medicine, particularly in cases of disappearances or cross-border crime.
- **Professional exchanges**: Exchange programmes enable forensic nurses to work abroad and gain international experience.

6. Technological developments and acceptance :

- **Adoption of new technologies**: While some countries are at the forefront of adopting new technologies, others may be resistant, whether for financial, cultural or legal reasons.
- **Data protection legislation**: Regulations vary considerably from country to country, impacting the way genetic or biometric data can be used and stored.

7. Ethics and professional conduct :

- **Codes of ethics**: Although many ethical principles are universal, certain aspects of forensic ethics may vary according to jurisdiction and culture.
- **Managing conflicts of interest**: The way in which conflicts of interest are identified and managed may vary from country to country, depending on their legal traditions.

Ultimately, although the science behind forensic medicine is universal, the way in which it is applied and interpreted is profoundly influenced by the local context. For the modern forensic nurse, navigating this international landscape requires both a solid scientific background and a nuanced understanding of the diverse cultures and legal systems with which they may interact.

The challenges posed by globalisation and mobility

As borders blur and populations move, forensic medicine must adapt to an ever-changing landscape. The challenges posed by globalisation and mobility affect many aspects of the discipline, from identification methods to ethical and legal issues.

1. Identification of persons :
   - **Multiple origins**: With the increased mobility of individuals, forensic nurses are increasingly confronted with victims of diverse ethnic and national origins.
   - **International databases**: The need to collaborate with foreign databases for identification purposes, in particular DNA, fingerprints and dental records, is increasing.
2. Legal challenges :
   - **Multiple jurisdictions**: Deaths occurring abroad or involving foreign citizens can pose challenges in terms of jurisdiction and applicable laws.
   - **Extradition and transfer of evidence**: The transmission of forensic evidence between countries can be complex, requiring judicial and diplomatic coordination.
3. Training and standards :
   - **Harmonisation of practices**: Globalisation calls for the standardisation of practices and standards in forensic medicine to guarantee uniform quality and ethics.

- **International training programmes**: Forensic nurses can benefit from training programmes abroad, while facing adaptation challenges.

4. Ethical and cultural issues :
- **Respect for beliefs and traditions**: Forensic nurses need to be aware of an increasing variety of funeral rites and religious beliefs.
- **Global human rights**: Human rights issues, particularly in areas of conflict or humanitarian crisis, require special attention.

5. Diseases and epidemics :
- **Emergence of new diseases**: Population mobility can introduce new diseases or conditions, altering the landscape of potential causes of death.
- **Epidemiological surveillance**: Identifying the causes of death during epidemics requires international collaboration and specific protocols.

6. Migration flows :
- **Identification of deceased migrants**: Tragedies involving migrants, such as drowning at sea, present unique identification and international coordination challenges.
- **Working with humanitarian organisations**: Organisations such as the Red Cross play an essential role in managing deaths during migratory crises.

7. International disaster management :
- **Interventions in disaster areas**: Forensic nurses may be called upon to work in areas affected by natural disasters or conflicts, requiring specific logistics and preparation.
- **Multinational collaboration**: These interventions often involve collaboration between experts from different countries, requiring effective coordination and communication.

Globalisation and the increasing mobility of populations offer both opportunities and challenges for forensic medicine. As techniques and technologies advance, forensic nurses must also evolve to meet the changing needs of a world on the move, while respecting the ethical and professional principles that are the foundation of their discipline.

Chapter 11:
COMMUNICATION
IN FORENSIC MEDICINE

Presentation of autopsy results
to families

Broaching the subject of autopsy with a bereaved family is a delicate task that requires great sensitivity, clear communication and deep respect for the loved ones of the deceased. The forensic nurse, who is often at the forefront of these exchanges, plays a central role in passing on information, allaying concerns and providing emotional support.

1. Preparing for the meeting :
   - **Full information**: Before meeting the family, the forensic nurse must be fully briefed on the details of the autopsy, the preliminary results and any procedures to be followed.
   - **Choice of setting**: Ideally, the meeting should take place in a quiet, private space that is conducive to discussion.
2. The empathic approach :
   - **Active listening**: It is essential to listen to the questions and concerns of loved ones before providing information. This allows the discussion to be tailored to their needs and knowledge.
   - **Acknowledging bereavement**: Giving importance to the emotions of families, acknowledging their pain and offering support.
3. Clear and transparent communication :
   - **Appropriate language**: Although medical jargon may be necessary, it is crucial to express yourself in simple terms that the family can understand.

- **Honesty**: If certain questions remain unanswered or if analyses are still underway, it is imperative that you say so.

4. Anticipating frequently asked questions :
   - **Reasons for an autopsy**: Families may wonder why an autopsy was necessary, especially if the death appeared natural.
   - **Autopsy procedures**: Briefly explain how an autopsy is carried out, while avoiding overly graphic details that could be upsetting.

5. Emotional support :
   - **Offer comfort**: A simple presence, a listening ear or words of consolation - any act of comfort can be precious.
   - **Referral to professionals**: If it becomes clear that the family needs additional support, the forensic nurse can refer them to psychologists or other professionals.

6. Confidentiality :
   - **Respect for personal data**: All information shared must remain confidential, in accordance with data protection laws.
   - **Discussion with the right people**: Make sure you only share the results with direct family members or authorised persons.

7. Next steps :
   - **Legal proceedings**: If the death is the subject of an inquest, inform the family of this process and what they can expect.
   - **Follow-up**: Suggest a later appointment to discuss the final results or to answer any further questions.

The presentation of autopsy results is a delicate but essential interaction. It provides an opportunity to provide answers, clarify misunderstandings and, above all, offer a measure of peace to grieving families. By approaching this task with empathy, professionalism and respect, the forensic nurse can provide invaluable support to those who need it most.

Communication of elements to the judicial authorities

Communicating forensic evidence to the judicial authorities is an essential part of forensic medicine. When correctly transmitted, this information can shed light on investigations, facilitate prosecutions or, conversely, exonerate the innocent. However, this communication must combine medical precision with judicial relevance.

1. Preparation of forensic reports :
   • **Clarity and precision**: Reports should be written concisely, avoiding unnecessary medical jargon, but with sufficient detail to be understood by non-specialists.
   • **Objectivity**: Conclusions must be based solely on the data collected, without subjective interpretation.
2. Working with the investigators :
   • **Regular exchanges**: Maintain fluid communication with interviewers to provide updates or answer their questions.
   • **Specific briefings**: In certain cases, specific briefing sessions can be organised to discuss key or complex elements of a case.
3. Presentation before the courts :
   • **Expert testimony**: As an expert, the forensic nurse may be called upon to testify in court to explain his or her findings and methodologies.
   • **Preparing for cross-examination**: Preparing for questions from defence lawyers who will seek to challenge or clarify certain conclusions.

4. Preservation of evidence :
- **Integrity of samples**: Ensure that all samples and evidence are properly stored, catalogued and preserved for future analysis.
- **Chain of custody**: Ensuring meticulous documentation of each stage in the collection, storage and transfer of samples to guarantee their legal validity.

5. Further training :
- **Updating legal knowledge**: It is crucial to keep abreast of legislative and regulatory developments that could affect the way forensic evidence is collected, stored and presented.
- **Interdisciplinary workshops**: Participating in training sessions with legal experts to better understand the expectations and needs of the legal system.

6. Ethics and professional conduct :
- **Confidentiality**: Only divulge information to authorised parties, while respecting the confidentiality of victims and families.
- **Professional integrity**: Avoiding any conflict of interest and ensuring that forensic work is always carried out impartially.

Communication between forensic professionals and the judicial authorities is a delicate dance that requires both solid medical expertise and sensitivity to the nuances of the legal system. By emphasising clarity, objectivity, ethics and collaboration, the forensic nurse can ensure that the forensic elements play their essential role in the administration of justice.

Report writing and official documents

Writing forensic reports is a complex and crucial exercise. These documents, which transcribe the observations and conclusions of the forensic nurse, are often central to legal proceedings. Rigorous, accurate and objective writing is therefore essential.

1. Understanding the importance of the report :
   - **Central document**: A well-written forensic report can influence the course of an investigation or trial.
   - **Legal liability**: Misrepresentations, whether intentional or not, can have serious legal consequences.
2. Structure of the report :
   - **Header**: Information about the forensic nurse, the forensic doctor in charge, the date and time of the examination, and details identifying the deceased or victim.
   - **Body of the report**: Detailed descriptions of observations, methodologies used and conclusions.
   - **Summary**: Summary of the main points and conclusions of the report.
3. Clarity and precision :
   - **Clear language**: Although the report is a medical document, it will be read by non-experts. The use of clear terms and the minimisation of jargon are therefore essential.
   - **Details**: Ensure the accuracy of descriptions, such as measurements, colours and positions.
4. Objectivity and impartiality :
   - **Factual basis**: Record only what has been directly observed or deduced from observations.
   - **Avoid speculation**: Do not include conjecture or personal opinions.

5. Confidentiality :
- **Sensitive information**: Personal details, such as names or addresses, should be treated with extreme caution and should only be included if necessary.
- **Secure storage**: Reports must be kept in a secure place to ensure data confidentiality.

6. Revisions and updates :
- **Proofreading**: Careful proofreading is required to ensure the accuracy and consistency of the report.
- **Updates**: If new information or analyses become available, the report should be updated accordingly, with clear documentation of the changes.

7. Transmission of the report :
- **Chain of custody**: Ensure accurate monitoring of report transmission to maintain its integrity.
- **Secure copies**: If copies are required, they must be correctly identified and stored.

8. Further training :
- **Writing workshops**: Specific training sessions can help hone writing skills.
- **Feedback**: Learn from previous cases and feedback from colleagues to improve the quality of future reports.

Writing reports and official documents in forensic medicine is a task that demands great responsibility, impeccable rigour and attention to detail. A well-written report not only testifies to the professionalism of the forensic nurse, but also plays a decisive role in the search for the truth in the judicial system.

Chapter 12:
PREVENTION AND AWARENESS

The nurse's role in prevention preventable injuries and deaths

Forensic medicine, despite its often post-mortem focus, has a crucial role to play in prevention. Forensic nurses, through their observations and expertise, can be agents of change to prevent avoidable trauma and death. This is a proactive role, involving both clinical and community action.

1. Trend analysis :
   - **Monitoring patterns** : By constantly observing the causes of death and trauma, nurses can identify trends or recurring patterns.
   - **Creating databases**: Gathering information to facilitate a broader analysis of the causes and circumstances surrounding incidents.
2. Awareness-raising and education :
   - **Prevention workshops**: Organising or taking part in information sessions aimed at educating the public about identified risks.
   - **Working with schools**: Working with schools to make young people aware of potential dangers and how to avoid them.
3. Interdisciplinary collaboration :
   - **Partnerships with the police**: Working with the police to implement preventive measures, such as speed checks or anti-alcohol campaigns.
   - **Involvement with social services**: Working together to prevent risk situations, such as mistreatment or abuse.

4. Participation in policy design :
- **Advice for decision-makers**: As experts in the field, forensic nurses can provide valuable information for developing public health and safety policies.
- **Advocacy**: campaigning for laws or regulations to reduce specific identified risks, such as improving road safety.

5. Continuing education and research :
- **Epidemiological studies**: Engaging in or supporting research to understand the root causes of preventable trauma and death.
- **Professional development**: Keeping abreast of best practice and new prevention methodologies.

6. Crisis intervention :
- **Psychological first aid**: Offering immediate support to people who have been traumatised or are in a crisis situation to prevent further damage or complications.
- **Referral**: Directing people to appropriate services, whether counsellors, rehabilitation centres or other health professionals.

7. Prevention in specific contexts :
- **High-risk environments**: Working in particularly vulnerable areas, such as neighbourhoods with high crime rates or conflict zones, to implement appropriate preventive measures.
- **Crisis situations**: Responding rapidly to major events, such as natural disasters or acts of terrorism, to minimise trauma and losses.

The role of the forensic nurse in preventing avoidable trauma and death is multidimensional. By combining clinical expertise, community awareness and political action, these professionals can make a significant contribution to the safety and well-being of individuals and communities.

Educating the public and raising awareness of forensic medicine issues

Forensic medicine, which is often shrouded in mystery and misunderstanding because of the way it is portrayed in the media, requires appropriate education for the general public. This awareness can not only inform, but also encourage closer collaboration between forensic medicine professionals and the community.

1. Demystifying forensic medicine :
   - **The difference between fiction and reality**: Clarifying the myths conveyed by TV series and films in relation to the reality of forensic work.
   - **Presentation of the different roles**: Explain the specific roles of forensic doctors, forensic nurses, technicians and other professionals.
2. Seminars and workshops :
   - **Interactive sessions**: Organising workshops for schools, universities and the general public on subjects such as the importance of autopsies, evidence collection and the chain of custody.
   - **Open days**: Invite the public to visit the forensic facilities to offer a hands-on perspective.
3. Working with the media :
   - **Articles and interviews**: Working with journalists to publish educational articles or give interviews clarifying certain aspects of forensic medicine.
   - **Documentaries**: Support the production of educational documentaries on the subject, offering an in-depth insight into the discipline.
4. Online resources :
   - **Dedicated websites**: Create and maintain websites containing reliable information, case studies and other relevant resources.

- **Webinars and online courses**: Offer virtual educational sessions to reach a wider audience.

5. Targeted awareness-raising :
- **At-risk groups**: Working specifically with communities or groups likely to be particularly affected by certain forensic cases, such as victims of violence.
- **Community partnerships**: Working with local organisations to co-organise events or information sessions.

6. Publications :
- **Brochures and leaflets**: Produce printed materials that are easily accessible to the public, explaining various aspects of forensic medicine.
- **Books and articles**: Encourage the publication of books aimed at the general public, detailing the realities of forensic work.

7. Raising awareness in emergency situations :
- **Responses to major incidents**: After events such as natural disasters, terrorist attacks or mass accidents, provide clear information on the medico-legal procedures underway.
- **Support for families**: Ensuring that victims' families understand the medico-legal process and their rights to information.

8. Integration into school curricula :
- **Science lessons**: Introduce the basics of forensic medicine into the school curriculum, particularly during biology or chemistry lessons.
- **Expert conferences**: Invite professionals to talk about their experience and work in educational institutions.

Educating the public and raising awareness of forensic issues is essential for building trust, dispelling myths and ensuring transparent collaboration with the community. It also serves to highlight the vital importance of this discipline, both for the justice system and for public health and safety.

Collaboration with organisations awareness and education

In the vast world of health, forensic medicine occupies a special niche, closely intertwining science, justice and emotion. The role of forensic nurses, as well as other professionals in the field, is poorly understood by much of the public. This is where collaboration with awareness-raising and educational organisations becomes crucial.

1. Identify potential partners :
   - **Health organisations**: Institutions such as the World Health Organisation (WHO) or ministries of health can provide a platform for educating the public about medico-legal issues.
   - **Specialist NGOs** : Many NGOs work to promote human rights, justice for victims of violence and medical science. They can be key partners in raising public awareness.
2. Joint awareness campaigns :
   - **Theme days**: Organise joint events, workshops and seminars on days dedicated to raising awareness of forensic issues.
   - **Educational material**: Co-create brochures, videos and web content to educate the public about forensic medicine.
3. Education and training :
   - **Joint training**: Offering training programmes for professionals and students, combining medical, legal and social expertise.
   - **School curricula**: Introduce forensic medicine into schools in partnership with education ministries, adapting the content to the level of the students.

4. Victim support :
- **Help centres**: Work with victim support organisations to provide clear information on forensic procedures and how they can help to achieve justice.
- **Testimonials**: Encourage forensic nurses and other professionals to share their experiences at events organised by victim support organisations.

5. Research and publications :
- **Joint studies**: Work with academic and research institutions to conduct studies on the effectiveness of forensic methods, victims' needs, etc.
- **Publications**: Co-editing articles, reports and books that shed light on collaboration between forensic medicine and other disciplines.

6. International projects :
- **Exchange programmes**: Creating opportunities for forensic nurses and other professionals to share their skills and knowledge abroad.
- **International workshops and conferences**: Organising joint events to discuss best practice and the challenges facing forensic medicine worldwide.

7. Online awareness :
- **Webinars and podcasts**: Organising virtual sessions to educate the public, using the combined expertise of forensic professionals and partner organisations.
- **Social networks**: Use platforms such as Twitter, Instagram and Facebook to share information and raise awareness of forensic issues.

In its quest for truth and justice, forensic medicine benefits greatly from collaboration with external organisations. By joining forces with bodies dedicated to education and awareness-raising, it not only raises its profile, but also increases the public's trust and understanding of it. This collaboration is therefore essential for establishing solid links between science, justice and the community.

Chapter 13:
FORENSIC MEDICINE RESEARCH

Importance of research
for the advancement of forensic medicine

Forensic medicine is a field where medicine, justice and forensic science meet. As an evolving discipline, it relies heavily on research to perfect its methods, refine its techniques and improve its protocols. Research in forensic medicine is therefore essential to guarantee the accuracy, reliability and relevance of its interventions. Let's find out how research shapes this field and why it is so crucial.

1. Refinement of autopsy techniques :
Research is helping to improve autopsy techniques, making these procedures less invasive while maintaining or even increasing their accuracy. This helps to extract essential information from the deceased with minimal disruption.

2. Advances in toxicology :
Toxicology is constantly evolving with the appearance of new substances, drugs and poisons. Research is used to identify these substances, develop more accurate detection tests and understand their effects on the body.

3. Advances in genetics :
Genetic research has revolutionised forensic science, with DNA sequencing enabling precise identifications. The evolution of this technology, including the use of environmental DNA or advanced genomic analysis, offers even more sophisticated tools for investigations.

4. Optimising the preservation of evidence :
The way in which evidence is collected, processed and stored is paramount. Research aims to ensure that

samples are not contaminated, degraded or otherwise compromised.

5. Improving identification methods :
Whether it's advanced imaging techniques, facial recognition or forensic anthropology, research is contributing to the development of ever more sophisticated methods of identifying victims, especially when traditional means prove ineffective.

6. Understanding decomposition phenomena :
By studying the various stages of decomposition in different environmental conditions, researchers can estimate the date and circumstances of death with greater precision.

7. Trauma assessment :
Research helps to better understand injuries and their causes, whether they result from accidents, violence or other events. This is crucial in determining the **exact circumstances of a death or assault.**

8. Interdisciplinary collaboration :
Forensic research is often enriched by collaboration with other disciplines such as psychology, anthropology, biology and chemistry. This multidisciplinary exchange promotes a holistic view of forensic cases.

9. Awareness-raising and training :
Forensic research also plays an educational role, enabling professionals to keep abreast of the latest advances, while training the next generation of nurses, forensic scientists and other experts.

10. Responding to contemporary social challenges :
In the face of crises such as pandemics, natural disasters or armed conflicts, research enables forensic methods to be adapted to specific contexts, guaranteeing relevant and effective interventions.

Forensic medicine is not simply a tool of justice; it is also a living, constantly evolving science. Without research, it would be static, unable to respond to the ever-changing challenges of our society. It is thanks to the tireless work of researchers that this field continues to illuminate the path to truth, offering clarity and resolution to those who desperately need it.

Involvement of the nurse in research projects

Nurses are often regarded as key players in patient care, but their role in research, although sometimes underestimated, is just as crucial. In forensic medicine, research is not limited to a distant academic activity; it is deeply rooted in the day-to-day reality of investigations and interventions. Nurses, as privileged witnesses of this reality, are ideally placed to contribute to the advancement of knowledge. Let's look at how and why nurses find themselves involved in forensic research projects.

1. The clinic as a source of observation :
Through their direct contact with forensic cases, nurses are often the first to identify anomalies, trends or unmet needs. These observations can lead to new research questions.
2. Participation in data collection :
Whether it's taking biological samples, physiological measurements or interviewing families, nurses are often on the front line when it comes to collecting accurate, reliable data.
3. Liaison role :
Nurses often act as a bridge between researchers and clinical reality. They can facilitate the implementation of research protocols, ensure compliance with ethical guidelines and guarantee the relevance of studies to clinical practice.
4. Application of findings :
Once the results of research are available, nurses are essential in implementing the new knowledge, by adapting

procedures, improving protocols or introducing new technologies.

5. Education and awareness :
Thanks to their central position, nurses can contribute to the continuing education of their colleagues, by sharing advances in research and ensuring that they are incorporated into daily practice.

6. Interdisciplinary collaboration :
Nurses can work closely with researchers from other disciplines, bringing their unique perspective and ensuring that the research is both **comprehensive and applicable.**

7. Development and evaluation of protocols :
As a medical professional, nurses have the necessary know-how to take an active part in developing new research protocols and evaluating their effectiveness.

8. Independent project management :
With the right training and experience, nurses can manage their own research projects, from conception to publication.

9. Publication and distribution :
Nurses involved in research projects may also contribute to the writing of scientific articles, the presentation of discoveries at conferences and the dissemination of knowledge within the forensic community.

10. A plea for research :
Based on their clinical experience, nurses can advocate more relevant research, identifying needs and mobilising the necessary resources.

Nurses' involvement in forensic medicine research projects strengthens the discipline itself. By combining clinical expertise, human sensitivity and scientific rigour, nurses help to advance the field towards ever more promising horizons.

Recent innovations
and their implications for practice

Constant advances in technology and research methodologies are shaping the landscape of forensic medicine. These innovations, while exciting, require professionals in the field, including forensic nurses, to continually adapt to maintain the relevance and effectiveness of their interventions. In this chapter, we explore the major innovations that have recently marked forensic medicine and their implications for everyday practice.

1. Advanced genomics and next-generation sequencing
These techniques have revolutionised the way in which biological samples are analysed. They offer unprecedented precision in identifying individuals and determining genetic links.
Implication: Better identification of victims, suspects or family members. This requires in-depth training to guarantee the integrity and validity of samples and analyses.

2. Non-invasive post-mortem imaging :
Techniques such as post-mortem MRI or CT scans offer a detailed view of the inside of the body without the need for an invasive autopsy.
Implication: Reduction in the need for invasive autopsies in certain situations, requiring specific training to correctly interpret the images and integrate them into the forensic process.

3. Improved toxicological analysis :
The ability to detect substances at extremely low concentrations, including new and unidentified drugs, has become a reality.
Implication: More precise identification of toxicity-related causes of death. This requires continuous updating of skills to keep pace with changes in the substances in circulation.

4. Virtual reality and 3D reconstruction :
These tools can be used to recreate crime scenes or events based on available evidence.
Implication: A better understanding of the events leading up to a death. Requires familiarity with software and technology.

5. Databases and artificial intelligence :
Advanced algorithms can now help identify trends, matches or anomalies in huge datasets.
Implication: Nurses can use these tools to improve their efficiency, but this requires an understanding of the basics of artificial intelligence and statistics.

6. Portable technologies for scene data collection :
Devices such as drones and portable scanners can be used to collect data on site.
Involvement: Greater autonomy in data collection, but training is needed to ensure the appropriate use of these technologies.

Innovations in forensic medicine are exciting, but they also bring their own challenges. For nurses, this means ongoing training, adaptability and a willingness to embrace change for the sake of science and justice. These tools, when used correctly, have the potential to significantly improve the accuracy, efficiency and impact of forensic medicine in society.

Chapter 14:
THE TECHNOLOGY
AND FORENSIC MEDICINE

The impact of new technologies
on forensic medicine

At the crossroads of technological advances and the relentless quest for the truth in matters of justice, forensic medicine is undergoing a revolution. These technological innovations have turned traditional practice on its head, bringing greater precision, unparalleled speed and possibilities that were once considered science fiction. Let's delve into the exploration of these technologies and their profound impact on the field of forensic medicine.

1. The digital age: digital forensics
With the emergence of the digital world, crime has also taken on a digital form. Extracting data from electronic devices, tracking digital footprints and detecting cybercrime have become essential.
Impact: This has broadened the scope of forensic science, making it a crucial element in the investigation of cybercrime and the detection of digital evidence.

2. Genomics and bioinformatics
Advances in DNA sequencing have made it possible to analyse ever smaller samples with unprecedented precision.
Impact: Unsolved cases from decades ago are now being answered, and the identification of victims in mass disasters is being speeded up.

3. 3D post-mortem imaging
The use of three-dimensional images to study cadavers, without the need for invasive cuts, is transforming autopsies.

Impact: More accurate studies of trauma, fewer intrusions into the body and greater acceptance by certain religious or cultural communities.

4. Artificial intelligence and machine learning

These technologies can analyse huge databases to detect patterns or correspondences that would escape the human eye.

Impact: Faster identification processes, improved facial recognition and prediction of criminal trends.

5. Drones and robots at crime scenes

These devices can access hard-to-reach areas, capture aerial images or even detect chemical substances.

Impact: Increased safety for investigators, wider coverage of crime scenes and more effective evidence gathering.

6. Augmented reality and virtual reality

Crime scene reconstruction, immersion in training environments or visualisation of events based on real evidence.

Impact: In-depth understanding of events, improved training for professionals and better presentation of evidence in court.

Technology is redefining forensic medicine, providing more accurate, rapid and extensive tools. However, with these advances comes the need for ongoing training, updated protocols and ethical reflection. Forensic medicine, while remaining rooted in its fundamental mission of seeking the truth, is evolving at breakneck speed, constantly pushing back the boundaries of what is possible.

Use of 3D modelling, virtual reality and artificial intelligence

Today's forensic medicine professionals have at their disposal cutting-edge technological tools that seem to have come straight out of a science fiction film. These technologies, ranging from 3D modelling to artificial intelligence, are revolutionising the sector. Let's take a closer look at the impact of these innovations on the world of forensic medicine.

1. 3D modelling :
Scanning and faithful reproduction of reality
- **Crime scenes:** Thanks to 3D modelling, a crime scene can be digitised and preserved indefinitely. Investigators can revisit the scene at will, without the risk of tampering with evidence.
- **Bone reconstructions:** For unidentified human remains, 3D modelling can be used to reconstruct a person's face and help with identification, particularly in cases that are several years old.

2. Virtual Reality (VR) :
Immersion and experience
- **Training professionals:** VR offers forensic nurses immersive training, putting them in real-life situations in a controlled environment.
- **Visualising autopsies:** Instead of carrying out a real dissection, some cases allow a "virtual autopsy", where the body is studied in detail using virtual reality images.
- **Court reconstructions:** Crime scenes or incidents can be reconstructed in VR for presentation in court, helping jurors to better understand the circumstances.

3. Artificial intelligence (AI) and machine learning:
Analysis and prediction
- **Pattern analysis:** AI can process massive amounts of data, spot trends and help deduce the likely causes of an incident or death.
- **Facial recognition:** Thanks to machine learning, systems can quickly identify an individual based on thousands of references.

- **Predicting crime trends:** With in-depth analysis, AI can also help to predict high-risk areas or crime trends, thus aiding prevention.

The convergence of these technologies in forensic medicine offers exciting and unparalleled opportunities for professionals in the field. However, with these innovations comes the ethical responsibility of their appropriate use. These tools, if used correctly, have the potential to take forensic medicine to an unprecedented level of efficiency and accuracy, benefiting both professionals and society as a whole.

Legal telemedicine : opportunities and challenges

Tele-medicine, a revolution in the delivery of remote healthcare through technology, has found its place within forensic medicine, giving rise to forensic tele-medicine. This merger enables health and justice professionals to interact, exchange information and provide services without being physically present in the same place. However, as with any innovation, it brings with it both promising opportunities and challenges.

Possibilities :
1. **Improved accessibility:** For remote areas or those without forensic experts, telemedicine can fill the gap, giving communities access to specialist skills and knowledge.
2. **Interdisciplinary collaboration:** This enables different experts (forensic doctors, nurses, investigators, lawyers) to collaborate in real time, regardless of their geographical location.

3. Training and education: Professionals can take part in remote training, seminars or consultations, improving their skills without having to travel.

4. Increased efficiency: Reports, analyses and consultations can be transmitted instantly, speeding up legal and medical processes.

Challenges :

1. Confidentiality issues: Transmitting sensitive data over networks can pose confidentiality and security problems. Ensuring encrypted and secure transmission is essential.

2. Validity of evidence: The quality of images or videos, or the perceived authenticity of remote information, could be challenged in court.

3. Technical limitations: Poor connection quality, network failures or technical faults can hamper the process.

4. Limited human interaction: Forensic telemedicine cannot always replace direct human contact, particularly for tasks requiring physical assessment or contact with a victim's next of kin.

5. Legal and regulatory framework: In many countries, regulation of telemedicine is still developing, and the question of its validity or recognition in the legal sphere remains a matter of debate.

6. Initial cost: Setting up a robust and secure technological infrastructure for forensic telemedicine may require significant investment.

Forensic tele-medicine has the potential to transform the forensic landscape, making services more accessible and processes more efficient. However, the successful adoption of this practice requires meticulous planning, investment in technology and an awareness of the ethical and legal implications. Only a balanced approach, which takes into account both the benefits and the challenges, will ensure its successful integration into the world of forensic medicine.

Chapter 15:
CAREER DEVELOPMENT
AND ADDITIONAL TRAINING

Possible specialisations
for the forensic nurse

Forensic medicine is a vast field offering a multitude of opportunities for nurses wishing to develop their skills and specialise. These specialisations enable nurses to play key roles in the collection, analysis and documentation of medical evidence in relation to the judicial system. Here are some possible specialisations for the forensic nurse:

1. Forensic nurse examiner (FNS) :
   - **Traumatology:** managing victims of violent trauma, documenting their injuries and collecting evidence.
   - **Examining crime scenes:** Helping to identify, document and collect forensic evidence.
2. Sexual Assault Nurse Examiner (SAEN) :
   - **Medical assessment:** Carrying out medical examinations on victims of sexual assault.
   - **Evidence gathering:** Ensuring the proper and secure gathering of evidence for later use in court.
3. Forensic psychiatric nurse :
   - **Psychiatric assessment:** Working with forensic psychiatrists to assess the mental state of people involved in legal proceedings.
   - **Tip:** Provide psychological support to victims or suspects.
4. Forensic toxicology nurse :
   - **Sampling:** Collecting samples for toxicological analysis.
   - **Interpretation:** To help determine the presence and effect of substances in an individual's system.

5. Paediatric forensic nurse :
  - **Child abuse:** Assessing and documenting signs of abuse or neglect.
  - **Education:** Raising community awareness of child trauma prevention.
6. Forensic nurse for the elderly :
  - **Elder abuse:** Identifying and documenting signs of elder abuse or neglect.
  - **Tip:** Provide support for elderly victims of crime.
7. Forensic anthropology nurse :
  - **Identification:** Helping to identify unidentified human remains.
  - **Documentation:** Working with anthropologists to document the characteristics and anomalies of the bones.
8. Thanatology nurse :
  - **Support:** Offering counselling services to bereaved families.
  - **Education:** Informing the community about the bereavement process and reactions to trauma.

By opting for one of these specialisations, nurses can not only enrich their careers, but also make a significant contribution to the justice and well-being of individuals and communities. These specialisations often require additional training and certification, but they open the door to rewarding and stimulating professional opportunities.

Complementary training and certifications

In the field of forensic medicine, nurses may need to undergo additional training and obtain certification to specialise or enhance their skills. This training and certification ensures competence, quality of care and better collaboration with other professionals in the field.

1. Additional training :
   - **Forensic science:** Furthering knowledge of the collection, preservation and analysis of evidence.
   - **Techniques for interviewing victims:** learning how to conduct sensitive interviews with victims in order to obtain information without causing them further trauma.
   - **Trauma assessment:** Specific training on the assessment of different forms of trauma, including injury, abuse and assault.
   - **Toxicology training:** Knowledge of toxic substances, symptoms of intoxication and sampling procedures.
   - **Forensic psychiatry:** Training on mental health assessment in a forensic context.
   - **Forensic anthropology:** training in the management and identification of human remains.
2. Certifications :
   - **IVEAS certification (Nurse Examiner of Victims of Sexual Assault):** A certification attesting to the nurse's competence in assessing and caring for victims of sexual assault.
   - **Certification in forensic sciences:** attests to the nurse's competence in collecting, preserving and analysing evidence.
   - **Certification in thanatology:** attests to nurses' skills in bereavement management and support for bereaved families.
   - **Certification in forensic psychiatry:** Attests to the nurse's skills in psychiatric assessment in a forensic context.
   - **Toxicology certification:** attests to the nurse's skills in the field of toxicology and toxicological analysis.

3. Workshops and seminars :
It is also recommended that forensic nurses regularly attend workshops, seminars and conferences to keep abreast of the latest advances, techniques and best practice in the field.

Continuing education and certification are essential for nurses wishing to specialise in forensic medicine. Not only do they ensure the quality of care and interventions, but they also reinforce the credibility and authority of nurses in this particularly sensitive field.

The importance of continually updating knowledge

Forensic medicine, like medicine in general, is constantly evolving. Scientific discoveries, technological innovations, new legislation and societal developments continually influence the way professionals in this field practice and interact with the justice system. For forensic nurses, continually updating their knowledge is not only beneficial, but essential for a number of reasons.

1. Ensuring precision and reliability :
Precision is crucial in forensic medicine. The conclusions of an autopsy or the analysis of samples can have major implications for the course of an investigation or trial. Obsolete or incorrect knowledge can have serious consequences, both for justice and for the people involved.
2. Maintaining professional relevance :
With the rapid evolution of techniques and tools, it is possible for certain skills to become obsolete. Continuous updating enables nurses to remain relevant in their field and to respond effectively to the changing demands of their profession.

3. Guaranteeing ethics and professional conduct :

New discoveries or techniques can raise ethical questions. A current and complete understanding of the issues enables nurses to make informed decisions that respect both the integrity of the individual and the standards of their profession.

4. Improving interprofessional collaboration :

Medical examiners, investigators, lawyers and other professionals depend on the information provided by forensic nurses. To facilitate smooth and efficient collaboration, it is crucial that the nurse is up to date with the latest practices and terminology.

5. Building trust :

The families of the deceased, the legal system and society in general place a great deal of trust in the skills of forensic nurses. By keeping their knowledge up to date, nurses reinforce this trust and ensure the credibility of their profession.

6. Anticipating and responding to challenges :

Whether faced with new drugs on the market, innovative methods of concealing evidence or societal challenges, up-to-date knowledge enables nurses to respond proactively.

Continuous updating of knowledge is not simply an option, but a necessity for forensic nurses. In a field where science, ethics and the law intersect, staying informed and competent is essential to ensure justice, respect for individuals and the integrity of the profession.

Conclusion
THE GROWING IMPORTANCE
OF THE FORENSIC NURSE

Over the years, the forensic nurse has gained greater visibility and recognition within the legal and medical system. From being a fully-fledged assistant to the forensic team, their role has evolved, revealing their crucial importance at every stage of the investigation and treatment. Let's take a look at why nurses have become key players in forensic medicine.

1. Clinical expertise :
The clinical skills of the nurse are essential, whether for the initial examination, taking samples or caring for the victims. Their medical expertise complements that of the forensic pathologist.

2. Raising awareness of victims' needs :
Nurses are trained in holistic patient care, which includes emotional and psychological aspects. This enables them to offer appropriate support to victims of violence or their families, while gathering the information needed for **the investigation.**

3. Mediation between disciplines :
The forensic nurse often plays the role of mediator between the various players involved in a case: doctors, police, families, lawyers. Their unique position enables them to facilitate communication and mutual understanding.

4. Managing complex situations :
Faced with delicate situations, such as the death of a child, the identification of a body after a disaster, or a case of extreme violence, nurses have the skills to manage these moments with humanity and professionalism.

5. Constant monitoring of procedures :
In a field where every detail counts, nurses ensure that protocols are followed to the letter, guaranteeing the integrity of the evidence and **information collected.**

6. Training and education :
Forensic nurses also have an educational role. They can train other professionals, help raise public awareness or contribute to **forensic science research.**

7. Technological adaptability :
With the rapid emergence of new technologies and methodologies, forensic nurses need to be at the cutting edge, adapting their practices and ensuring that they are implemented correctly.

8. Ethics and professional conduct :
Nurses, by virtue of their training and professional oath, are guarantors of ethical principles, ensuring respect for the deceased, victims and their families.

The forensic nurse is no longer on the sidelines, but at the heart of the system. Their contribution guarantees not only the quality and precision of forensic interventions, but also the humanity and ethics that are essential in this field. With the constant challenges and developments in forensic medicine, the role of the nurse is set to become even more important, demonstrating the crucial importance of the link between justice, medicine and society.

The need for a multidisciplinary, collaborative approach

Forensic medicine, although deeply rooted in the medical world, cannot function in isolation. It lies at the intersection of many fields - legal, psychological, social and scientific, to name but a few. The interweaving of these disciplines requires close collaboration between different professionals to ensure optimal care for victims, a full investigation and fair justice. Understanding the importance of such multidisciplinary collaboration is essential to grasping the complexity and depth of forensic medicine.

1. Complementary expertise :
Each professional brings a specific perspective and expertise. The nurse can detect subtle clinical signs, the forensic pathologist has an in-depth knowledge of pathology, the psychologist assesses emotional trauma, while the police officer investigates the criminal background. Together, they form a complete picture.

2. Quality of evidence :
The integrity of evidence is crucial to the judicial system. Close collaboration between professionals ensures that evidence is collected, preserved and analysed according to strict standards.

3. Holistic support for victims :
Victims of crime, particularly the most violent, need comprehensive care. A multidisciplinary approach meets their medical, psychological, social and legal needs.

4. Smooth communication :
Collaboration encourages transparent and fluid communication between disciplines. This avoids misunderstandings, speeds up investigations and ensures that all parties are well informed.

5. Cross-disciplinary education and training :
Collaboration also encourages the exchange of knowledge between disciplines. Nurses can learn more about the legal aspects of cases, while investigators can be trained in the clinical intricacies.

6. Changes in practices :
Faced with new challenges - such as the emergence of new drugs or new criminal methods - a multidisciplinary team can adapt more quickly and develop innovative responses.

7. Informed decision-making :
With the input of different experts, decisions taken, whether in the context of an investigation or treatment, are better balanced and based on an overall view.

In an increasingly complex world, where the boundaries between disciplines are increasingly blurred, a multidisciplinary approach in forensic medicine is not only desirable, it is essential. It ensures that each case is treated with the rigour, compassion and thoroughness it deserves, while valuing the contribution of every professional involved. Ultimately, it strengthens public confidence in the judicial and medical system.

Future prospects for the sector

Forensic medicine, like all other medical fields, is constantly evolving. Technological, scientific, socio-cultural and legal advances are constantly shaping and redefining this landscape. As nurses and healthcare professionals, it is crucial to understand these emerging trends if we are to stay at the cutting edge of the discipline, respond appropriately to the issues of the day and anticipate the challenges of tomorrow.

1. Personalizing forensic medicine :
Advances in genomics and biotechnology are making it possible to offer more targeted analyses. We can look forward to an era when forensic medicine will be more precise, identifying not only a cause of death, but also genetic predispositions or underlying pathologies.
2. The rise of technology :
Virtual and augmented reality, 3D modelling, artificial intelligence and robotics will transform the way autopsies and analyses are conducted. These technologies will

enable more accurate reconstructions of crime scenes or incidents, helping to solve complex cases.

3. Ethics in the digital age :

With the increasing digitisation of forensic data, the issues of confidentiality, data security and ethics will grow in importance. Professionals will be faced with unprecedented dilemmas concerning the use, storage and sharing of this data.

4. A global reach :

Globalisation and the increasing mobility of populations pose challenges in terms of identification, especially in the event of major disasters or massive migratory movements. The interconnection of databases and international collaboration will become essential.

5. A renewed focus on mental health :

Growing awareness of the importance of mental health will highlight the need to provide support not only for the families of the deceased, but also for the professionals who deal with death on a daily basis.

6. Continuing education and training :

The increasing complexity of the discipline will require more specialised training. Forensic nurses may have to undergo more advanced training, perhaps even obtaining specialist degrees.

7. The expanded role of the forensic nurse :

With better training and increasing recognition of their expertise, it is likely that nurses will play a more central role in medico-legal proceedings, perhaps even becoming forensic experts in their own right.

The future prospects for forensic medicine are vast and stimulating. For nurses prepared to embrace these changes, the opportunities for professional growth, innovation and societal impact are immense. While some of these changes may seem daunting, they also offer a chance to improve and refine the discipline, making it even more essential to modern society. The key will be to remain adaptable, informed and always ready to learn.

Glossary of forensic terms

- **Forensic anthropology**: Scientific study of human remains in a legal context, often used to determine the identity of unknown bones.
- **Asphyxia**: Lack of oxygen leading to respiratory failure, often examined as a cause of death.
- **Autopsy:** Post-mortem examination of a body to determine the cause of death.
- **Ballistics**: Study of projectiles, often used in forensic medicine to analyse gunshot wounds.
- **Corpse**: Dead body, especially when referring to a deceased person.
- **Contusion**: injury to the skin caused by an impact, without breaking the skin.
- **Cyanosis**: Blue discolouration of the skin due to insufficient oxygenation of the blood.
- **Decomposition:** Process by which the body decomposes after death.
- **Forensic entomology**: Study of insects in connection with a criminal investigation, often used to estimate the time of death.
- **Exhumation:** The act of removing a body from its grave for medico-legal reasons.
- **Haematoma**: Accumulation of blood in a tissue following an injury.
- **Incision:** A cut or wound caused by a sharp object.
- **Laceration**: Irregular wound caused by a tear in the tissue.
- **Forensic pathologist: a** doctor who specialises in determining the cause of death.
- **Suspicious death**: Death occurring in unusual or unexpected circumstances, requiring investigation.
- **Necrosis**: Death of organic tissue.
- **Forensic odonatology**: Study of teeth to identify a corpse.

- **Pathology**: Study of diseases and their causes.
- **Rigor mortis**: Rigor mortis that occurs after death.
- **Forensic toxicology**: Study of poisons, drugs and other toxic substances and their effects on the body.
- **Traumatology**: Study of injuries and their effects on the body.
- **Victim**: A person who has suffered harm, injury or death as a result of a criminal or accidental act.
- **Interpersonal violence**: Violent acts committed between two or more individuals.
- **Yersinia pestis**: Bacterium responsible for plague, often studied in forensic medicine in the context of identifying ancient remains.

This glossary is of course not exhaustive. The field of forensic medicine is vast, and many other terms are used regularly by professionals in the field.

Resources and professional associations

Forensic medicine, like the nursing profession within it, is supported by a solid network of organisations and resources that work to provide training, professional support and research. Here is an overview of the main resources and associations that play a crucial role for forensic nurses.

- Professional associations
  - **Association Internationale des Infirmiers Médico-légaux (AIIML) (International Association of Forensic Nurses):** An organisation that brings together nurses specialising in forensic medicine from all over the world. It offers training courses, conferences and specialist publications.
  - **Société de Médecine Légale et de Criminologie de France (SMLCF):** Although it encompasses a wider range of professionals, this society plays an important role in training and networking for nurses in France.
  - **Association des Médecins Légistes d'Expression Française (AMLEF):** facilitates exchanges between professionals and promotes research in forensic medicine.
- Newspapers and publications
  - **Journal de Médecine Légale:** Publishes research, case studies and literature reviews which may be particularly useful for nurses seeking to keep abreast of the latest developments.
  - **Forensic Science International:** A world reference in the field of forensic medicine.

- **Forensic Nursing:** Focusing specifically on the role of nurses in this field, this journal covers both clinical practice and research.
- Training and certification
  - **Certificate in forensic medicine for nurses**: Many universities and nursing schools offer specific training courses to specialise in forensic medicine.
  - **Ongoing training**: Training modules, seminars and webinars are regularly organised to enable nurses to update their skills.
- Online resources
  - **ForensicNurses.org**: An international portal dedicated to forensic nurses, with resources, forums and news from the field.
  - **MedLeg.fr:** French-language website containing information, articles and resources for forensic medicine professionals.
- Trade fairs and conferences
  - Events such as the **International Congress of Forensic Medicine** provide opportunities for nurses to meet experts, learn and share experiences.
- Psychological support and well-being
  - Many associations recognise the emotional and psychological challenges faced by forensic nurses and offer resources, training and support on wellbeing and stress management.

By becoming actively involved in these organisations and using these resources, nurses can not only improve their professional skills, but also contribute to the evolution and recognition of the crucial role of nurses in the field of forensic medicine.

Bibliography and recommended reading

The field of forensic medicine, and in particular the role of nurses within it, is vast and constantly evolving. Here is a non-exhaustive list of essential references to help you learn more about the subject:

- General works on forensic medicine:
  - **Madea, B.** (Ed.). *Handbook of Forensic Medicine*. John Wiley & Sons. A comprehensive work on forensic medicine, covering everything from pathology to toxicology.
  - **Vinchon, M., & Gosset, D.** (Eds.). *Traité de médecine légale*. Elsevier Masson. A French-language reference work dealing in depth with the various aspects of forensic medicine.
- Forensic nurses:
  - **Lynch, V. A., & Duval, J. B..** *Forensic Nursing Science*. Elsevier Health Sciences. This book, although written in English, is a comprehensive guide to forensic nursing practice.
  - **Hammer, R. M., Moynihan, B., & Pagliaro, E. M..** *Forensic Nursing: A Handbook for Practice*. Jones & Bartlett Learning. Another major reference for nurses interested in forensic nursing.
- Psychological and support aspects:
  - **Stevens, M..** *Forensic Nursing and Multidisciplinary Care of the Mentally Disordered Offender*. Jessica Kingsley Publishers. This book explores the role of nurses working with mentally disordered offenders.
- Autopsy and post-mortem procedures:
  - **Burton, J. L., & Rutty, G. N..** *The Hospital Autopsy: A Manual of Fundamental Autopsy*

Practice. CRC Press. A comprehensive guide to hospital autopsy relevant to forensic nurses.
- Toxicology and analysis:
  - **Karch, S. B.**. *Pathology & Toxicology of Drug Abuse*. CRC Press. A detailed exploration of the effects of drugs and toxic substances on the human body.
- International forensic medicine:
  - **Ubelaker, D. H.**. *Handbook of Forensic Anthropology and Archaeology*. Routledge. For those interested in forensic science in an international context, this book offers an anthropological perspective.
- Specialist newspapers and articles:
  - Don't forget to check the latest editions of forensic journals for recent case studies, research and journal articles.
- Resources on ethics in forensic medicine:
  - **Gurley, L. R.**. *Ethics in Forensic Science*. Academic Press. A book that delves into the ethical dilemmas and considerations facing forensic science professionals.

Each of these readings offers unique perspectives and valuable information for anyone wishing to deepen their knowledge of forensic medicine, whether as a specialist nurse or simply for information purposes. It is always advisable to check availability in university libraries, specialist bookshops or online platforms.

www.ingramcontent.com/pod-product-compliance
Lightning Source LLC
Chambersburg PA
CBHW062331290526
45794CB00005B/1986